52
ways
to
walk

ALSO BY ANNABEL STREETS

*The Age-Well Project: Easy Ways to a Longer, Healthier,
Happier Life* (with Susan Saunders)

(WRITING AS ANNABEL ABBS)

NONFICTION

Windswept: Walking the Paths of Trailblazing Women

FICTION

The Joyce Girl

Frieda: The Original Lady Chatterley

Miss Eliza's English Kitchen

52

The Surprising Science of Walking for Wellness and Joy, One Week at a Time

ways
to
walk

Annabel Streets

G. P. PUTNAM'S SONS | NEW YORK

PUTNAM
— EST. 1838 —

G. P. Putnam's Sons
Publishers Since 1838
An imprint of Penguin Random House LLC
penguinrandomhouse.com

Library of Congress Cataloging-in-Publication Data

Names: Streets, Annabel, author.
Title: 52 ways to walk: the surprising science of walking for wellness and joy, one week at a time / Annabel Streets. Other titles: Fifty-two ways to walk
Description: New York: G. P. Putnam's Sons, 2022. |
Includes bibliographical references and index.
Identifiers: LCCN 2021053561 (print) | LCCN 2021053562 (ebook) |
ISBN 9780593419953 (Hardcover) | ISBN 9780593419960 (eBook)
Subjects: LCSH: Walking. | Walking—Research.
Classification: LCC GV199.5 .S78 2022 (print) |
LCC GV199.5 (ebook) | DDC 796.51—dc23/eng/20211112
LC record available at https://lccn.loc.gov/2021053561
LC ebook record available at https://lccn.loc.gov/2021053562

Printed in the United States of America
1st Printing

Book design by Lorie Pagnozzi
Illustrations by Alexis Seabrook

FOR HUGO

contents

5²
ways
to
walk

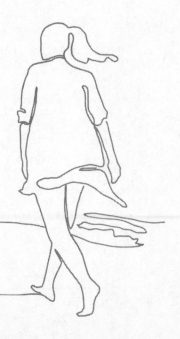

introduction

WHEN I WAS TWENTY-THREE AND had a little money in my pocket, I learned to drive and bought a small, rattling car. I loved my car, often driving around town for the sheer thrill of it. You see, I grew up carless. My father never owned a car; he never even learned to drive. My mother finally took lessons in her forties, proudly failing her driving test seven times. We lived in obscure, remote places where public transport was at best unpredictable, and at worst non-existent. If we needed anything, we walked, often for miles and miles. Perhaps this explains why my little Fiat brought me such pleasure.

My driving life coincided with a desk job. Both eventually coincided with curious changes to my body (rounder, softer, achier, stiffer, stooped) and to my mind (anxious, unsettled, discontented). Around the same time, I came across a fact that flabbergasted me. I read—in Bill Bryson's *A Walk in the Woods*—that the average American walked 1.4 miles a week.

In that instant I saw how dramatically my life had changed. Because I was no better—hopping into my car at every opportunity, slouched over a desk all day, slumped on the sofa all evening. Suddenly I had a deep yearning for the life I'd lost, with its simple walking joys, its endless adventures on foot, its wild blustering air. I decided to "upmove" my life, to reoxygenate it.

I made a rule for myself: not to use my car unless it was absolutely necessary. Instead, I would walk. During the months that followed, I noticed that many of the journeys I'd taken by car were ridiculously close to home. Why had I driven to a supermarket that was only a twenty-minute walk? To a dentist that was a mere fifteen-minute saunter? More ludicrous still, why on earth had I driven to a gym so that I could walk on a treadmill or sit on an exercise bike?

I noticed something else too: at the first sign of rain, wind, darkness, heat, hunger, boredom, lack of a companion—to name a paltry few of my many excuses—my little car became irresistibly alluring. And so I bought a dog and proper wet-weather clothing—no longer would the cold, wet, or dark excuse me from walking. I grew to love my night walks, my rain-sodden strolls and mud-bound marches, my after-dinner ambles, my windy weekend hill hikes, and my ley-line saunters. Walking had never seemed more beguiling or more thrilling.

Later—and while suffering from debilitating, desk-induced back pain—I made a second rule-for-self: to convert as many of my sedentary activities as possible into walking activities. Work would be walked, holidays would be on foot, the weekly shop would be militarily *rucked*, coffee with a friend would become a strolling coffee . . . Only to hear the same excuses I'd once given myself. Colleagues turned down my invitations to bipedal meetings: too windy/hot/cold/early/late. Friends (some) and family (especially) were no different: too far/steep/muddy/heavy/boring . . . especially boring.

A question began gnawing at me: What if all these excuses were, paradoxically, good reasons *to* walk? By this point, I was regularly researching and writing about the subjects of walking and health. Studies on the astonishing power of movement and nature—sunlight, soil, snow, silence, scent—were tumbling into my in-box, confirming some of my recent suspicions. I began my own series of walking experiments: hiking at altitude, in forests, barefoot, and backward; walking by moonlight; following rivers, pilgrim routes, fractals, or my own nose; dancing and singing as I strode; litter picking, forage walking, mindful walking, power walking, silent walking . . . Walking had become, once again, the great adventure of my life. But this time science could explain how and why.

Meanwhile, reports of its impact on health seemed incontrovertible. Regular walking was helping millions of people to reverse diabetes, fend off heart disease, hold back cancer, lower blood pressure, reduce weight, counter depression and anxiety—and so much more. Indeed, one study concluded that exercise was preventing almost 4 million premature deaths every year, a figure deemed conservative by some epidemiologists, who believe walking could avoid up to 8 million deaths a year. Another study claimed that thirty-five chronic diseases could be prevented by exercise.

Because here's the thing: when we move, hundreds of intricate changes take place inside our bodies. A twelve-minute walk alters 522 metabolites in our blood—molecules that affect the beating of our heart, the breath in our lungs, the neurons in our brain. When we walk, oxygen rushes through us, affecting our vital organs, our memory, creativity, mood, our capacity to think. Walking causes hundreds of muscles, joints, bones, and tendons to move in an elaborate, effortless sequence, propelling us forward but also triggering a multitude of molecular pathways, expanding our heart, strengthening our muscles, smoothing the lining of our arteries, shunting sugar from our blood, and switching our genes on and off in a miraculous process known as epigenetic modification. Walking does more than enrich our own health. It also enriches the health of future generations. We know that exercising in our reproductive years produces children who are more resistant to disease; we know that *active* pregnant women produce a compound in their breast milk that reduces their babies' lifelong risk of diabetes, heart disease, and obesity.

Moreover, every time we choose to walk, we reduce the burden of air pollution and noise pollution. We prevent yet more land being turned over to concrete parking lots and out-of-town shopping centers. Every time we petition our governments and city councils to create walkable routes and parks, to protect woodlands and wetlands, we help build a better world for everyone, now and into the future. Walking in nature brings us closer to the land, making us care more about it—from its tiny insects and lichens to the grandeur of its mountains and trees. And when we care about something, we want to conserve it. Right now, our spectacular world needs conserving.

And what of our towns and cities? They too deserve to be walked. They too are enriched when we stride them rather than drive them—cleaner, more convivial, quieter, safer.

We have driven (literally) walking out of our lives. And yet we were born to walk. Not only for a few minutes on pleasantly sunny days in cushioned sneakers following a Google dot, but in drenching rain and squalls of wind, uphill and downhill, in winter and at night, alone and in crowds, in forests and beside rivers, in search of food and in pursuit of smell, even backward and barefoot.

It's time to rethink walking, to reclaim it from our molecular memories. Walking is not—and has never been—boring. We might be stuck in a walking rut: same route, same time of day, same companion. But there are hundreds of ways to walk and hundreds of reasons for doing so. And many routes can be taken directly from our front door, wherever we live or work, immersing us instantly in a magical tangle of wildlife, geography, geology, astronomy, history, culture, and architecture.

Nor is walking merely step-counting or "exercise." Yes, good physical and mental health are happy by-products. But the joys of walking are infinitely greater than clocking up steps. Think of it as a means of unraveling towns and cities, of connecting with nature, of bonding with our dogs, of fostering friendships, of finding faith and freedom, of giving the finger to air-polluting traffic, of nurturing our sense of smell, of satisfying our cravings for starlight and darkness, of helping us appreciate the exquisitely complicated and beautiful world we inhabit.

I hope this book spurs you to rediscover the delight, mystery, wonder, and exhilaration of walking. I hope that—through its fifty-two ways to walk—you too will find bipedalism endlessly interesting, perpetually rewarding. Lastly, I very much hope you enjoy the bounteous happiness and health that always, always, accompany a lifetime of walking.

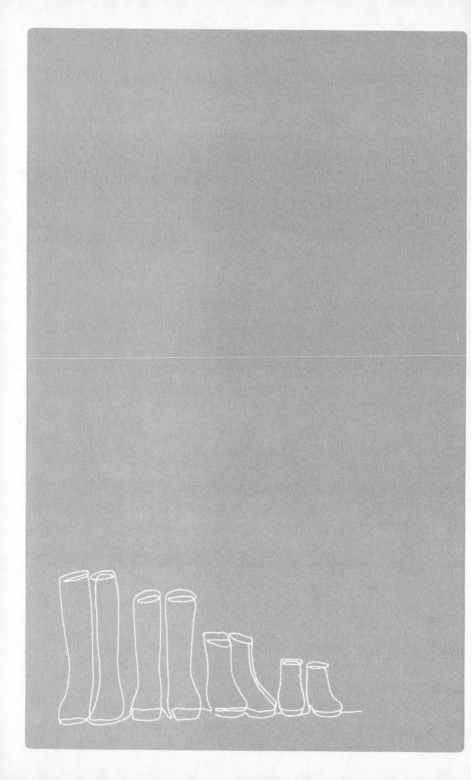

How to Use This Book

EACH CHAPTER IN THIS BOOK is an opportunity to try a new mode of walking, and for this reason I've arranged it over a calendar year, week by week. I've attempted to match chapters with weather conditions, or—on occasion—with universally recognized "events." More importantly, I've arranged it to be dipped into, according to your circumstances and desires, much like a buffet breakfast bar. It's my fervent hope that by experimenting with different walking styles, timings, weather conditions, routes, and locations, you'll keep discovering something novel, unexpected, revelatory, even.

We think of walking as being splendidly spontaneous—something we can do as and when we want without any planning or forethought. This is, of course, one of the great joys of walking. We can step out of our house and just go.

But the unexpected and the revelatory are, paradoxically, more likely to occur if we start with a little preparation and planning. Racing out to enjoy a wet wintry walk is infinitely easier if we have the right kit—and know where to find it. A moonlit amble is more enjoyable if we have a route, a full moon, a friend, and the right footwear. Going out to sketch is well-nigh impossible if we have neither sketchpad nor pencil. Besides, research shows that the most consistent walkers are more likely to have a walking schedule than those who simply nip out for a stroll. So before you dip in and dash out, get organized: that means checking kit and making a rough plan.

Investigate maps, books, apps, and online sites for new paths, pilgrim routes, long-distance trails, nearby ley lines, unexplored tracks, enticing destinations, and so on, jotting down any you like alongside projected timings (allow an hour to walk two miles) and transport, parking, and eating options.

A few walks in this book require a kit. Night hikes, mountain treks, and wet-weather walking (for example) are more enjoyable taken in comfort. And that means having the right gear in good working order.

The best way to check the quality of your waterproofs (boots, parka, *and* rain pants) is to wear them in the shower. If they leak, run them through the washing machine with a quality wash-in waterproofer. Clean and waterproof your walking boots, replacing the laces if necessary.

For urban walking, you'll want comfortable shoes. For me, that means a sneaker with a wide, square toe box; a slim, flexible sole; and a zero-drop heel design, which means toe and heel are at the same height. Shoes that are too small risk numbing and swelling feet by cutting off blood flow, while oversize shoes can lead to stumbling and tripping. So experiment to find the footwear that best suits you.

If you're walking in your regular sneakers, check they're not worn down. Studies show that aging athletic shoes can affect posture and gait, ultimately leading to potential injuries. If you're concerned about falling, choose a lightweight, laces-free shoe with a nonslip rubber outsole designed to provide extra grip. Whatever you walk in, make sure it's comfortable, breathable, and waterproof if need be.

For longer hikes, or treks over rugged terrain, you'll need a stout (broken-in) walking boot with a rugged sole and ankle support. And hiking socks—quick-drying, breathable, anti-blister (if you're prone to blisters). I have hiking socks for both summer and winter, bought at end-of-season sales.

If you're intending to do day hikes and want to be ready to leave at a moment's notice, keep a small backpack ready. I keep mine stocked with a few blister bandages and antiseptic wipes, a package of tissues and a couple of painkillers, a water bottle, a small sketchpad with pencil and eraser, a lightweight set of binoculars, sunscreen, a Shewee, and a packet of nuts.

Keep your strolling kit (sunglasses, sunscreen, hat, gloves, umbrella, parka, door keys, portable coffee cup, water bottle, insect repellent, whatever you need) in a single, easily accessible place so that you're ready to seize the sunlight, the moonlight, or a rainstorm.

For winter hikes and wind walks, thermal layers, gloves, hat, and thick socks are essential, while a thermos is a bonus. For long-distance walks, consider a pair of telescopic walking poles—particularly if descents are involved—and make sure your backpack is comfortable.

Providing children with their own (small) backpacks containing their favorite snacks cuts down on complaints, carrying, coaxing, and cajoling.

If you're planning to walk in areas with Lyme disease, keep insect repellent in your pack.

For quick local walks, pockets or a fanny pack enable you to keep your skeleton aligned, your posture perfect, and your arms swinging.

With your pack ready and your ramshackle plan pinned to the wall, you're all set to go. No need to scroll through trail maps or bus timetables, or search for missing parkas, water bottles, or blister bandages. Instead, pick a week and get reading. Nothing on Netflix? Turn to Week 42 (p. 173) and swap your screen for a health-enhancing after-dinner stroll. Having trouble sleeping? Take a look at Week 50 (p. 207) and discover how to walk for deeper sleep. Inclement weather deterring you from walking? Turn to Week 12 (p. 48) and explore the mind-boggling benefits of walking in rain. Eyes dry and aching from too much computer time? Turn to Week 8 (p. 33) on the miracle of panoramic vision as you ramble. Too tired to walk? Take a peek at Week 4 (p. 18), where I investigate the rousing advantages of a slow stroll. You get the idea . . .

And then get up, get out, get walking!

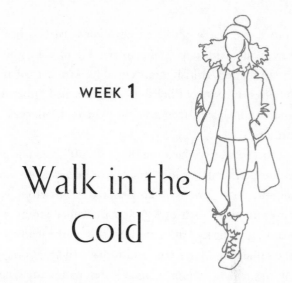

Walk in the Cold

THE EIGHTEENTH-CENTURY WALKER AND WRITER Elizabeth Carter claimed her favorite walks were those taken in "whistling winds and driving snows." Carter wasn't as unusual as we might think. Over the years, hundreds of walkers have expressed an enduring love for ice-blasted walks in the glacial depths of winter. In Christiane Ritter's astounding account of living in the Arctic Circle, she describes her daily walk in temperatures of −31°F: "I take my walk every day . . . in circles, ten times, twenty times, over the uneven snow drifts that have frozen as hard as steel." Walking to Lhasa in 1924, the explorer Alexandra David-Néel (who famously mastered the ancient meditative practice of *thumo reskiang* to self-heat) was stunned into enthralled silence by "the immensity of snow . . . an everlasting immaculate whiteness." Later, having trudged through miles of knee-high snow, she pronounced it "paradise."

And yet for many of us, winter is the time we chose *not* to walk, preferring to stay home in the warm and dry. Big mistake! Decades after Carter, Ritter, and David-Néel embraced the cold, scientists are finally disentangling the extraordinary changes that take place in our bodies and brains when we spend time in *moderate* cold. Of course, ice, snow, and cold have been used to heal for centuries: Egyptian manuscripts refer to the use of cold water for reducing inflammation, British monks used ice as a form of anesthetic, and a nineteenth-century English physician called James Arnott used salt and crushed ice to reduce the pain of headaches and cancerous tumors.

Fast-forward to Japan in the year 2000, and one of the first modern experiments to hint at the complexities of cold. Researchers identified two groups of female walkers: one group wore long skirts, covering every inch of leg, and the other group wore miniskirts, exposing their legs from ankle to thigh. The women agreed to wear the same skirts for a year and to have their legs regularly scanned. At the end of winter, magnetic resonance imaging (MRI) scans revealed that the legs of the miniskirted women had acquired an extra layer of fat. The legs of the long-skirted women, however, remained unchanged. This doesn't mean that exposure to cold makes us fat. Quite the reverse—as scientists were about to uncover.

At the time it was thought that only hibernating mammals and babies carried a protective wrapping of brown fat, despite emerging studies implying that a few adults (outdoor workers in Scandinavia, for example) might also have pockets of it secreted beneath their skin. It was to be another decade before American researchers discovered the remarkable truth about brown fat—sometimes called brown adipose tissue (BAT)—the cold-induced fat acquired by the Japanese miniskirt wearers.

In spite of its unfortunate name, brown fat is entirely free of the harmful lipids associated with excessive white or yellow fat. In fact, brown fat is a more effective fat burner than anything else, including muscle tissue, which might explain why thin, active people often carry more brown fat than their larger, more sedentary counterparts.

But the most dramatic discovery came when researchers analyzed brown fat and found it packed with mitochondria, the tiny factories inside our cells that convert the food we eat and the oxygen we breathe into a form of energy called adenosine triphosphate (ATP). ATP supports every cellular process in our body. Brown fat exists to keep us warm and breathing (alive), which explains why a flash of cold spurs it into life—increasing our metabolism, regulating our appetite, improving our insulin sensitivity, halting the premature death of our cells.

Brown fat achieves this by producing molecules called batokines, which help preserve us in multiple ways. For example, batokines appear to stimulate production of follistatin, a protein that strengthens our muscles. Batokines also increase a compound called IGF-1, which encourages growth in every cell we have, meaning (very simply) that our bodies are better able to repair themselves, and hinting at why a 2021 study found people with good stocks of brown fat were also less likely to suffer from hypertension, congestive heart failure, and coronary artery disease. No wonder scientists are hopping with excitement at the therapeutic possibilities of brown fat.

Not only does brisk walking in cold weather keep our cells healthy and our bodies in trim, muscular shape, it also keeps our brains in good working order. Studies suggest that we think more clearly in cold weather than in hot weather. Our brains run on glucose, and when glucose is low, our brains become sluggish. We use more glucose cooling down than we use warming up, which could explain why some of us feel brain-foggy in hot climates but zingily alert in cold climates. A 2017 study from Stanford University found that people thought more decisively, calmly, and rationally in lower temperatures than in higher temperatures, reflecting a 2012 study that found warm weather not only impaired people's ability to make complex decisions but made them more reluctant to engage with the decision in the first place.

We don't need to *feel* cold to experience enhanced cognition: merely *looking* at "cold" pictures makes our brains work with greater rigor. When Israeli researchers gave people a series of cognition tests interspersed with background images of either wintry, summery, or neutral landscapes, the participants achieved their best scores when they had the wintry images in their peripheral vision.

Cold, in moderation, is also good for our mental health. A study of Polish students found that fifteen minutes in a chilly, leafless forest had "substantial emotional, restorative and revitalizing effects," implying that nature can make us feel just as rejuvenated in bare winter as in green-gold spring.

Finally, a spot of cold appears to reduce feelings of stress. A 2018 report from the University of Luxembourg found that repeatedly applying cold to the necks of volunteers activated their parasympathetic (calming) nervous system, slowing and steadying heart rates—and raising the possibility that a judicious dose of chill could be more calming than one might think.

None of this is to suggest we purposefully make ourselves cold and miserable. Instead, we should welcome the colder months as an exhilarating time to walk. The views are altered: Who doesn't love the new vistas through sculpturally skeletal trees? Or the monochrome geometry of lines and shapes? Birdlife is more readily visible. Our brains are sharper, more zestily alert. Our beneficial brown fat is urged into action. To top it all, we build endurance: in lower temperatures, our hearts don't have to work so hard and we sweat less, meaning our bodies work more efficiently.

TIPS

HOW COLD DOES IT HAVE to be? Not particularly . . . Brown fat is activated in mild cold, around 61°F, according to Dutch physiologist and brown-fat researcher Wouter van Marken Lichtenbelt.

How long should we walk for? As long as suits, but one study found that two hours of exposure to moderate cold triggered the conversion of (bad) white fat (particularly in our stomachs and thighs) into (good) brown fat.

Hate the cold? Numerous studies show that cold becomes less intimidating and discomforting the more we expose ourselves to it—a process called habituation. Wrap up warmly and increase the length of your walks bit by bit.

Worried that cold air exacerbates allergies and asthma? A growing body of evidence suggests that winter exercise may do quite the reverse, reducing allergic inflammation in the airways and improving respiratory symptoms in many adult cases.

Wear layers, so that you're neither too hot nor too cold. Hands, feet, and head are often the first to cool, as blood floods to our vital organs to keep them warm, so wear fleece-lined gloves, thick socks, and a hat. If you're warm enough, expose your forearms for vitamin D and your neck to activate brown fat (which often lies under the skin of the neck and collarbones, according to Ronald Kahn, professor of medicine at Harvard Medical School).

Take a flask of something hot. We often get unknowingly dehydrated in cold weather.

A flask of coffee will help activate our brown fat: caffeine, like exercise and cold weather, is thought to spur brown-fat production.

Walking in deep snow can be exhausting, so consider snowshoeing—an excellent way to walk long distances through snow.

Worried about slipping on ice? Ensure your footwear has the best possible grip/traction (check sites like ratemytreads.com). Walk slowly and sideways on steps and downhill. Use walking poles. Our arms help us balance and our hands can prevent falls, so keep your gloved hands out of your pockets.

The cold is not a panacea, and hypothermia can kill, so wear the right clothes and footwear and walk as energetically as you can (see Week 2: Improve Your Gait, p. 10).

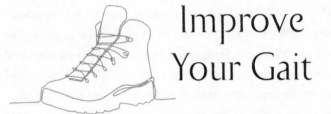

Improve Your Gait

WHEN A YOUTHFUL ADMIRER TOLD the French philosopher Simone de Beauvoir that he liked the way she walked, it was a compliment she never forgot. How we walk—our gait—provides a window into who and *how* we are. After Canadian researchers observed 500 walkers, they were able to identify (with an impressive 70 percent accuracy rate) which walkers had early cognitive impairment, reflecting previous studies suggesting that our gait at the age of forty-five can predict our chances of getting Alzheimer's. Merely by observing gait, explained Manuel Montero-Odasso—an expert in the relationship between mobility and cognitive decline—we "can help diagnose different types of neurodegenerative conditions." In other words, how we walk reflects how well our brain is functioning, hinting at what the future might have in store for us.

Scientists don't yet know whether changes in our brain affect our gait or whether changes in our gait affect our brain. Either way, we need to pay attention to the way in which we walk. And yet how many of us do this? Putting one foot in front of the other, propelling ourselves forward, is the simplest and most natural of movements— one we master as toddlers. But it's also an act of unimagined complexity, involving balance, coordination, strength, and the firing of hundreds of neurons. When we walk, we engage almost every muscle and bone we possess, all of them synchronized in an extraordinary sequence of moves that no machine has ever been able to replicate.

Our indoor laptop lifestyle is making it harder for us to walk with the effortless efficiency and grace of our forebears. Our bodies have lost much of their strength, balance, and suppleness, thanks to feet squeezed into fashionable shoes, days stooped over laptops, and evenings spent lolling on sofas. Meanwhile, our feet tilt, totter, and plod, their 159 bones, muscles, and joints barely used.

Does this really matter? Arguably, yes. A poor gait compromises how we move, meaning we aren't experiencing the full freedom (and pleasure) that accompanies a smooth, flowing stride. Nor are we enjoying the full physiological benefits. Sports scientist Joanna Hall believes our current lifestyles are detrimental to *how* we walk. Sitting for too long has shortened and tightened our hip flexor muscles and encouraged our stomachs to slump. Crouching over desks and laptops has forced our necks and heads to jut unnaturally forward, stiffening our spines and restricting our back muscles. Leaning forward, for hour after hour, has weakened the small postural muscles that control the curve of our spines, leading to lower back pain.

Meanwhile, walking in the wrong shoes has cramped our toes and stiffened the muscles in our feet so that we strike the ground with a flat plod (which Hall calls a *passive foot strike*) rather than a springy rolling sole (an *active foot strike*). And hitting the ground without using the splayed spread of our feet risks misaligning our pelvis. "We need to learn how to use the right muscles in the right way at the right time," she tells me as she puts my own walking style to rights.

Hall—who has spent the last twenty-five years helping people walk as their bodies intended—recommends relearning how to walk in order to avoid injury and joint strain, and to enable us to pick up our speed and walk for longer. Research carried out by London South Bank University found that a month of walking with a full range of motion resulted in an accelerated walking speed and improved skeletal alignment. Hall's advice includes:

- Pushing off from the back foot, using the muscles at the backs of our legs.
- Peeling through each foot from heel to toe, using all of our toes to drive us forward.
- Lifting our ribs and lower spine to activate our abdominal muscles and create space in our core.
- Lengthening and straightening our neck, which frees our spine to move as we walk, while counteracting the stiffness that comes from long hours hunched over a computer.
- Swinging our arms freely from the shoulders, using our elbows to impel us forward—not in the manner of a 1980s power walker, but more as if our arms were a pair of smoothly jointed pendulums. Our hands should be loose, not bunched into fists.

Medics at Harvard Medical School advise looking ten to twenty feet in front of you and lowering your eyes rather than your head when you need to check the ground (an upright head reduces the chance of neck pain). They also recommend swiveling the hips very slightly, saying "a slight pivot can add power to our stride," and taking care not to overstretch our stride, adding "concentrate on taking shorter steps but more of them."

Of course you can walk in your own way, adjusting nothing. But, according to Hall, "getting our gait right reduces the chance of stiffness in our joints and spine." Harvard Medical School echoes this, saying that poor ingrained walking habits can be easily reversed ("with a little work") to avoid injury, to make walking both more beneficial for our health and more enjoyable.

Getting our gait right means we can walk faster, should we want to. All walking is good—and in some circumstances slow walking is better (see Week 4: Just One Slow Walk, p. 18, and Week 42: Walk After Eating, p. 173)—but several studies suggest that brisk walking, around 4 miles per hour (or 100 to 130 steps per minute), brings extra benefits. A 2019 study found that brisk walkers lived longer than slower walkers, concluding that a faster pace meant "a lower risk of a wide range of important health conditions." Walking at a good clip means all our daily exercise can be accommodated as we walk to school, to work, or to the shops.

Improving our gait also means we can walk for longer periods of time. Studies suggest that longer bouts of walking are particularly good for reducing body fat and improving mood. When we can walk effortlessly for hour upon hour, our opportunities for walking expand. We can hike long distance (see Week 36: Walk with a Pack, p. 148), walk pilgrimages (see Week 40: Walk Like a Pilgrim, p. 165), follow a river from source to sea (see Week 17: Follow a River, p. 67), or simply *walk* a route that we previously *drove*.

But there's another reason for relearning how to walk. When we move in alignment, with the spring and grace our bodies were built for, we also feel happier and more certain of ourselves, as if the newfound lightness in our limbs has crept into our minds, loosening us from our everyday cares and constraints.

TIPS

CONSIDER YOUR OWN WALKING STYLE, making any adjustments and practicing the suggestions above, taking them one by one. You should feel lighter and more upright, with a slightly accelerated pace.

Ask a friend to check your gait, posture, and alignment, or video yourself walking and make your own assessment.

Remember that your footwear affects your gait. Invest in comfortable, low-heeled shoes that fit properly and are appropriate for your intended walking.

Bags also affect gait. Opt for a backpack, fanny pack, or belt bag.

Walking poles can help with posture and gait. Try a pair of hiking poles, adjusted to your height.

If you need help with your gait, look for walking coaches or online tutorials.

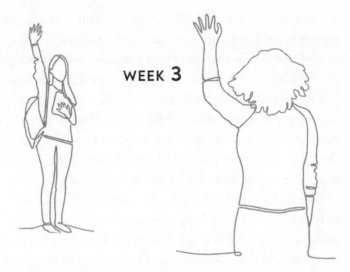

WEEK 3

Walk, Smile, Greet, Repeat

IN 2005, THE BRITISH PSYCHOLOGIST Dr. Cliff Arnall declared Monday of the third week of January to be the saddest day of the year. A combination of bad weather, dark nights, failed new-year resolutions, and post-Christmas debt culminated—he claimed—in a day of universal and collective depression: "Blue Monday."

Arnall urged us to think ahead to holiday time. I think a neighborhood walk would be more effective. Walking exposes us to chance encounters with other people. Greeting others—neighbors or strangers—with a smile improves how we feel, both in mind and body, ensuring we return home happy rather than snappy, gracious rather than grumpy. We don't need to exchange words—a smile is sufficient.

For several years psychologists speculated that the simple act of smiling could transform our mood, although they weren't sure how or why. They used the phrase "fake it to make it," reminding us that even a cheesy sculpted smile could lift our sense of well-being.

A 2020 study from the University of South Australia confirmed that simply smiling (however forced) can trick the mind into feeling more upbeat. Participants were asked to hold a pen between their teeth, nudging their facial muscles into the semblance of a smile. Apparently, when we forcefully practice smiling, our brain is stimulated into releasing neurotransmitters that make us feel more positive—which is exactly what happened to the participants of this study, who reported not only feeling more cheerful but perceiving things around them—including other people—as also more cheerful. Their forced smile effectively changed the lens through which they viewed the world.

I don't like to think of this exercise as faking or forcing a smile, but rather as activating a smile. When we activate a smile, a neurological reaction takes place that lifts our mood and makes everything seem less foreboding. Although an activated smile feels a little artificial at first, my own experiments suggest that it doesn't take long before it feels entirely natural. Exchanging smiles with passersby is one of the fastest ways to transition an activated smile into a genuine smile. And these human exchanges in turn help raise our mood a little higher. Studies by the psychologist Eric Wesselmann have found these brief moments of connection to be profoundly important, helping us feel we belong. In Wesselmann's studies, participants who were recognized by others (with a smile, nod, or even an exchange of eye contact) reported greater self-esteem than those who were ignored.

Other studies have found that people who've received greetings feel more encouraged to smile at and greet others, a sort of cascade effect that can help an entire swath of us start our day with a little more buoyancy and hope.

Smiling (or walking with a pencil between your teeth if you must) isn't the only way to shake off a grumbling mood or a lurking bleakness. Other studies have found that participants who adjusted their body posture or introduced new gestures became, for example, more confident or more determined. A 2009 study from Ohio State University found that when people improved their posture, they were more inclined to believe in themselves, while a 2018 study from San Francisco State University found that students with upright posture performed better in math tests than slumped students.

Walking, greeting, and smiling does more than lift our own mood. As Antonia Malchik explains in her seminal book *A Walking Life*, noticing and greeting others as we stroll is one of the ways in which human beings have historically built social capital. Passing exchanges while on foot is one of the richly sticky threads that successfully weaves a community together. And study after study shows the importance of community to our well-being—Blue Monday or otherwise.

TIPS

ALWAYS PUT YOUR PERSONAL SAFETY first. Only ever greet or smile at strangers when you're sure it can't be misconstrued. Early morning dog walkers are famously friendly (and usually safe).

Once comfortable, turn up the corners of your mouth, step out, greet passersby with a broad smile—and walk away from crankiness, doubt, disappointment, defeat . . .

The walking techniques in Week 2: Improve Your Gait (p. 10) will give you the confidence to smile and greet. Shoulders back, standing tall, chin raised, arms swinging—and for exactly the same reason: our body is tricking and triggering our brain into releasing mood-boosting neurotransmitters.

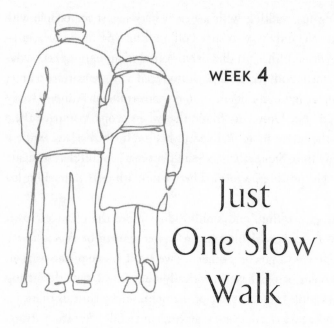

WEEK **4**

Just
One Slow
Walk

TWO YEARS AGO, I BROKE a bone in my foot. After an X-ray at
my local hospital, I was dispatched to sit at home with my leg raised.
I bought a pile of books and settled in for a few weeks on the sofa.
A few days later the orthopedic consultant called me, wanting to
know how my walking was progressing. "Walking?" I spluttered
into the phone. "I can't possibly walk!" Calmly and with complete
certainty, she told me to get up, strap on my orthopedic clog, and
start walking. "Just one slow walk . . ." she said, explaining that I
could use crutches or a stick, take frequent rests, and move as slowly
as I wanted. But the actual walking was non-negotiable. "See it as a
treat," she added. "How often do we give ourselves permission to
walk slowly?"

Although brisk walking is the most lauded walking style for
overall health, a slow walk can often be as effective. Recent studies
suggest that a slow walk every day—even one with plenty of rests—

can have powerful long-term effects, and not just for people with broken bones.

When American researchers found that mouse pups with active mothers were healthier in later life than mouse pups with sedentary mothers, they decided to replicate the experiment with humans. Using activity trackers, they followed 150 women through pregnancy and early motherhood. Regular testing of breast milk revealed that the more steps a mother took, the more abundantly she produced a compound called 3'-SL (oligosaccharide 3'-sialyllactose). It's thought that consuming milk rich in 3'-SL reduces a baby's lifelong odds of developing diabetes, heart disease, and obesity. Other reports suggest that plenty of 3'-SL also improves a baby's future capacity to learn, focus, and remember. But what most surprised the researchers was how unimportant exercise *intensity* was. A slow daily walk was enough to trigger the production of 3'-SL in the mothers' milk.

For older people who find walking more difficult, research suggests that rather than hang up their walking boots, they should adapt and modify their walking technique. A study followed 36,000 adults over the age of forty for nearly six years, with a team of scientists recording the amount, type, and frequency of exercise taken by each individual. The results showed that any level of activity, regardless of intensity, was associated with "a substantially lower risk of death." All it took was one slow walk a day.

Sports scientists believe that perseverance is vital and that almost anyone can manage a slow walk—whether you're heavily pregnant, in your nineties, or recovering from injury. The key is to modify your style of walking. Researchers in Finland found that older people who continued to walk long distances but used walking sticks, a slower pace, and frequent rests along the way were more independent and had better mental and physical health than those who stopped walking, believing it had become too demanding or difficult.

We know that sitting for as little as an hour cuts blood flow through the legs to the heart by as much as 50 percent, affecting cholesterol levels and jeopardizing our heart and metabolic health. But American researchers say that a slow five-minute walk every hour reverses the damage. When the researchers asked a group of men to move for five minutes every hour at a speed of two miles per hour, their extended sitting ceased being detrimental to their heart health. "Light physical activity can help," concluded the research team.

A team from Maastricht University found similar results when it conducted an experiment on eighteen students. Those who walked for the longest amount of time but at slow speeds had significantly lower cholesterol and triglycerides, and healthier insulin levels, than students who cycled like crazy for an hour but then spent the rest of their day at a desk. Long, slow walks may be better than short, high-intensity runs, speculated Professor Hans Savelberg, adding that the most important thing is to reduce our time spent sitting. Other studies have suggested that if we're overweight, long, slow walks may be better for us, burning more calories and putting less pressure on our joints—one study revealed that walking at a leisurely 2 mph rather than a brisk 3 to 4 mph reduced the load on knee joints by up to 25 percent. Another study of midlifers found that a leisurely 8,000 steps a day meant "a dramatic difference in whether you live or die," according to Dr. Edward Phillips at Harvard Medical School. In a nutshell, distance—at any pace and with any number of rests—surpasses intensity.

Of course, the quiet, unhurried serenity of a gentle stroll makes it more conducive to many other things, from generating new ideas, to after-dinner digestion (see Week 42: Walk After Eating, p. 173). This might be because slow walking allows us to engage paced breathing—deep slow breaths from the diaphragm taken at half our normal rate of breathing (roughly seven breaths a minute). Paced breathing is not only calming but proven to lower heart rate and blood pressure. Suzanne LeBlang, a neuroradiologist who has investigated paced breathing, suggests it stimulates the vagus nerve, which then reduces stress chemicals in the brain, relaxing and widening the muscle cells lining our veins and arteries—and enabling our blood to flow more freely.

TIPS

IF YOU'RE WALKING SLOWLY AS part of a rehabilitation program, always check with your doctor first, and choose smooth, even surfaces.

Avoid polluted areas and busy roads, particularly if the traffic is slow-moving. Pollution has been linked to an ever-lengthening list of conditions, from Alzheimer's and Parkinson's to asthma and death from COVID-19, with more being added as research intensifies.

Walk amid greenery. A study of 20,000 people found those who spent two hours a week in green spaces, either on a single walk or spaced over several, were substantially more likely to report good mental and physical health. There were no benefits for people spending less than two hours a week.

Rather than disparage your own slowing pace and diminishing distance, remember the words of writer and walker Clara Vyvyan: "A walk of two miles can be as rich and rewarding as a walk of twenty miles."

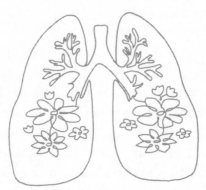

Breathe as You Walk

THE EIGHTEENTH-CENTURY GERMAN PHILOSOPHER Immanuel Kant famously walked every day at five P.M. He was such a stickler for routine that the inhabitants of his town, Königsberg, used to set their clocks as he walked past. But Kant was attentive to more than his timekeeping. Obsessed with notions of health, he was fascinated by his breathing. In fact, Kant developed a technique of breathing solely through his nose—250 years before scientists recognized the role of nasal breathing for good health. Kant was so determined to breathe only through his nose that he refused to walk with a companion, fearful that conversation might inadvertently make him inhale through his mouth. Kant lived to just short of his eightieth birthday, a phenomenal age in 1804.

Nasal breathing is often associated with a deep sense of relaxation, but scientists now believe the physiological benefits of "in through the nose, out through the mouth/nose" breathing go well beyond feelings of serenity. Walking is the perfect time to hone your breathing. So take a stroll—and breathe through your nose.

Why? Because when we inhale through our nose, a series of intricate processes takes place designed to filter out airborne pathogens, allergens, and other undesirables. Meanwhile, our nasal cavities produce nitric oxide (NO), which increases blood flow through the lungs, building up the amount of oxygen in our blood. When we inhale through our mouths, not only do we bypass the remarkable filtering system offered by our nose, but we also deprive our cells of the additional oxygen offered by nose breathing, because the mouth produces no nitric oxide.

From our nose, nitric oxide moves directly into our lungs, where, according to pharmacologists, it can block viral respiratory infections that replicate in the lungs (such as coronaviruses), as well as boost the flow of oxygen and blood through our bodies.

Nitric oxide is an extraordinary molecule, produced constantly by the cells lining our arteries and veins (known as endothelial cells). Discovered in our bodies a mere thirty-five years ago, when scientists spotted its role in dilating blood vessels, nitric oxide helps prevent high blood pressure and blood clots and pushes blood through to our vital tissues and organs. It also plays a part in maintaining immunity, in keeping our nervous system healthy, and in slowing the cellular aging process. In fact, malfunctioning nitric oxide has been linked to both Parkinson's and Alzheimer's diseases. When it comes to aging, nitric oxide plays a very particular role in helping cells to survive for longer. Indeed, the complex machinations of nitric oxide are only just being understood.

During the 2002–4 SARS outbreaks and the COVID-19 pandemic, researchers speculated that nitric oxide might stop the spread of some viruses in the lungs. Studies confirmed that they had speculated correctly. One revealed that patients with pneumonia were more likely to make a good recovery if they inhaled nitric oxide. Another found that mouth breathers had lower levels of nitric oxide in their respiratory tracts and were more likely to suffer from heart disease, fatigue, inflammation, headaches, stress, halitosis, and tooth decay (among other things). The researchers wondered if the extra nitric oxide generated by nasal breathing might reduce the viral load on our bodies, giving our immune systems a better chance of successfully fighting back.

Delivered directly into our lungs (by nose breathing), nitric oxide seems to help fend off attack from microorganisms and viruses. According to Professor Louis Ignarro, one of the three pharmacologists who won the 1998 Nobel Prize for uncovering the workings of nitric oxide, we need to "practice breathing properly to maximize the inhalation of nitric oxide into our lungs" by inhaling through our noses, where nitric oxide is continuously produced.

Nose breathing also appears to improve our general health and fitness. A recent study found that we breathe more slowly when we inhale through the nose, creating extra time for oxygen to enter our bloodstream and helping to activate parts of the nervous system supporting recovery. In his book *Breath: The New Science of a Lost Art*, James Nestor makes the full case for nasal breathing, arguing that it lowers blood pressure, aids sleep, eases digestion, builds bone, and may even improve our brains. His own experiments of mouth versus nose inhalation while exercising revealed that nasal breathing as we move improves endurance and reduces subsequent fatigue, while mouth breathing resulted in exhaustion, nausea, and bad breath.

As you walk, close your mouth; relax the jaw, tongue, and face; and breathe slowly in through the nose and out through the mouth. You'll find this more challenging as your pace picks up. But stay focused and you might—possibly—have fewer colds, more energy, and greater serenity.

According to Nestor, optimal health derives from breathing correctly—slow and deep, with an in-breath duration of 5:5 seconds followed by an out breath of the same duration—resulting in a mathematically satisfying 5:5 breaths a minute.

TIPS

WANT TO TAKE YOUR NASAL breathing further? Try humming as you walk. One study found that humming resulted in an oscillating airflow into the nose that yielded significantly greater amounts of nitric oxide. Indeed, hummers produced *fifteen times* as much nitric oxide as regular breathers.

Ensure your posture is perfect: lengthening your neck and opening your chest and shoulders will encourage more proficient breathing.

Take a tissue. In cold weather, nasal breathing can leave noses prone to running.

Nasal breathing also allows us to receive the full effects of scent and smell (see Week 11: Take a City Smell Walk, p. 44, and Week 39: Walk with Your Nose, p. 161).

Finally, nasal breathing is a vital part of the best technique I know for long uphill hikes (see Week 35: Walk Like a Nomad, p. 144).

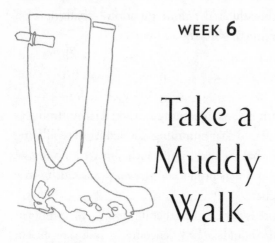

Take a Muddy Walk

MUD AND SODDEN EARTH OFTEN deter us from going for a walk. Fearful of slipping or of getting cold, wet feet, we avoid mud-bound paths in favor of tarmac. But instead of treating turned and open soil as a reason for *not* walking, we should see it as the reverse—a reason to step out, to choose the soggy path in preference to the asphalt path, and to breathe deeply as we do so.

Ever since penicillin was cultivated from a soil fungus, scientists have been investigating the health and healing properties of Earth. In 2015, researchers at Northeastern University announced a newly tested antibiotic produced from soil that kills resistant strains of staphylococcus and tuberculosis. Other discoveries followed: researchers have been working on a soil microbe called *Mycobacterium vaccae*, which—in the brains of mice—produces the feel-good hormone serotonin, thereby acting as an antidepressant. A study done at Russell Sage College in Troy, New York, showed that mice fed *M. vaccae* in miniature peanut-butter sandwiches had less anxiety, were more efficient at learning new things, and ran through mazes with both greater speed and greater competence. As the authors explained to *New Scientist*, the *M. vaccae* mice navigated the maze twice as fast and exhibited half of the anxiety behaviors of those that didn't consume the bacterium.

The mood-enhancing effects of this soil bacteria were discovered accidentally by a London oncologist, Professor Mary O'Brien, who created a serum out of the bacteria and gave it to lung-cancer patients, hoping it might boost their immune systems. Instead, she noticed another effect: the hospital patients cheered up. They reported feeling happier and suffering from less pain than the patients not receiving doses of the bacterium. Curiously, they also reported greater levels of energy and an ability to think more lucidly.

A researcher at Bristol University tested Professor O'Brien's results by injecting mice with the bacterium, speculating that it triggered the mouse brain to make serotonin. His experiment revealed that the mice injected with *M. vaccae* were calmer than those that didn't receive an injection of the bacterium.

Gardeners responded with great enthusiasm. They had always known that working with soil was a powerful mood enhancer. The researchers, however, speculated that soil-induced serotonin did more than blunt feelings of anxiety: it also aided concentration. "From our study we can definitely say it is good to be outdoors . . . to have contact with these organisms," they wrote. "Time in the outdoors where *M. vaccae* is present may decrease anxiety and improve the ability to learn new tasks."

Being in the presence of mud and soil may also be good for our gut. An experiment carried out by Australian researchers found that mice exposed to good-quality soil had more diverse microbiomes and less anxiety than a control group exposed to either poor soil or no soil. Importantly, the "quality soil" mice microbiomes had abundant butyrate. One of the best-researched and most desirable of microbiota, butyrate is being investigated for its anticancer and anti-inflammatory properties. Soil (particularly when it comes from a forest floor) produces a bacterium that, once ingested, makes butyrate in our gut, prompting suggestions that exposure to biodiverse soils could be good for both gut and mental health.

Mud and soil exposure, particularly in areas of farmland, might also help reduce the risk of asthma. According to Dr. Helen Cox, one of the UK's leading pediatricians specializing in allergies, several studies—including one in *The New England Journal of Medicine*—have linked the lower rates of asthma in farm-raised children to the wide diversity of bacteria in their living environment.

Meanwhile, a substance known as geosmin, derived from bacteria and found in wet earth, is known to induce feelings of calm. We are deeply sensitive to this rich smell, able to detect the equivalent of seven drops of it in a swimming pool. Evolutionary psychologists think we find the smell of geosmin calming and reassuring because it alerted our distant ancestors to the presence of water and fertile soil. Geosmin was the smell of survival.

The evidence is clear: not only should we relish the chance to walk through earthy and muddy landscapes, but we might also want to plunge our hands in at some point, fill our lungs with the scent of soil, and not be too assiduous when we wash it off.

Still not convinced of the miracle of mud? Walking in mud—or on any unstable surface like gravel, shingle, marsh, or cobblestones—is superb for our balance. As we tip and tilt, the twenty-nine different muscles in our core work hard to ready and steady us, keeping us strong, stable, and balanced.

TIPS

TRY SMELLING AND TOUCHING THE damp land on your route: the leafy soil of forest floors, the damp sands of a beach, the muddy shores of a river.

Prod small patches with a stick to help release geosmin.

Still hankering for asphalt? Stick with mud: recent research found that sunlight and rain cause an ingredient in asphalt to leach thousands of potentially toxic compounds into the environment.

Worried about slipping and sliding? Take walking poles or use your arms for balance, and rest assured that every lurching step is improving your spatial awareness, balance, and core muscles.

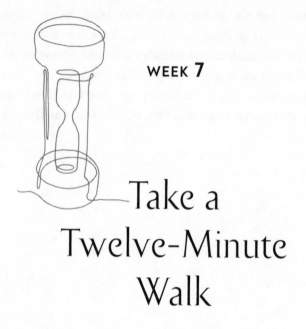

Take a Twelve-Minute Walk

WE ALL HAVE DAYS WHEN finding the time for a walk seems impossible. In the weeks after my father died suddenly and unexpectedly of a heart attack, I found myself either frantically busy or utterly exhausted. The idea of a walk seemed ridiculously ambitious. And yet it's during these times of overwhelming indoor busyness and emotional fatigue that we most need to move. Grief, like stress, alters the body, provoking inflammation, reducing immunity, and putting us at greater risk of heart disease. As I grieved, slumped, and feverishly organized—a peculiarly toxic blend of activity and inactivity—a study from Massachusetts General Hospital dropped into my in-box, motivating me to nip out for a (very short) walk.

The study suggested that I didn't need to walk for hours: twelve minutes was sufficient to dramatically impact my health. Hospital researchers had studied 411 middle-aged men and women, measuring the levels of 588 metabolites circulating in their blood. By measuring these—a process known as metabolite profiling—before and after exercise, the researchers could determine not only the manner in which exercise affected each metabolite, but the amount of exercise required before those changes took effect.

Metabolites are small molecules that reveal how well (or not) our bodies are functioning and how effectively our cells are repairing themselves. Doctors use metabolites as biological markers to gauge what's going on inside us and to check our metabolic health and the current state of our heart, among other things.

The researchers in this study found that, after twelve minutes of brisk walking, over 80 percent of these remarkably revealing biomarkers had changed for the better. One of these changed metabolites was glutamate: we all have glutamate lurking inside us, pumped out by our brains when we're exposed to stress and toxins. Too much circulating glutamate is a biomarker for heart disease, diabetes, and a shorter life span. Excessive glutamate has also been linked to a paucity of brain cells, which is to say too much glutamate might play a role in brain shrinkage. The researchers found that twelve minutes of exercise typically lowered glutamate levels by 29 percent. Meanwhile, a metabolite associated with liver disease and diabetes dropped by 18 percent, and a metabolite known to break down fat stores rose by 33 percent.

"What was striking to us was the effects a brief bout of exercise can have on the circulating levels of metabolites that govern such key bodily functions as insulin resistance, oxidative stress, vascular reactivity, inflammation and longevity," explained study author Gregory Lewis in *Men's Health* magazine. Lewis is also section head of the heart failure unit at Massachusetts General Hospital, so I took note. Not only had my father recently died of sudden heart failure, but in my grief-stricken nights I often felt such clenched pain in my chest I thought that I too was on the verge of a heart attack.

It seemed to me that for anyone in the throes of grief, a daily walk was more essential than ever. And so I began urging myself out, ignoring the mounting paperwork and my endless cravings for the sofa. There was only one issue: this study made it clear that my walk had to be "vigorous" or "intense" rather than a dawdling stroll. Brisk or uphill walking, where our heart rate is accelerated, making us a little breathless and sweaty, is ideal. I found a twelve-minute route and walked it once a day, as fast as I could.

TIPS

UNSURE WHAT BRISK MEANS? AIM for 100 plus steps in a minute. Set the timer on your phone for sixty seconds and count each step until you get to a hundred. If the timer goes off before you've done a hundred steps, try picking up your pace.

Unable to walk fast? Build your speed by including brief bursts of acceleration (Harvard fitness consultant Michele Stanten recommends fifteen-, thirty-, or sixty-second bursts) before returning to your normal pace for one to two minutes. Repeat.

Walking with the right gait will help you pick up pace. Practice the postural and foot-strike techniques suggested in Week 2: Improve Your Gait (p. 10).

Time a twelve-minute route from your door so that—on exceptionally busy days—you don't need to think about anything other than putting on your shoes.

Anyone can find twelve minutes. If your days are too crowded, consider a short, sharp night walk (see Week 46: Take a Night Walk, p. 190) or a prebreakfast yomp (see Week 10: Walk Within an Hour of Waking, p. 40).

Got more time? Studies suggest that a few short walks are better for lowering blood pressure than a single longer walk, particularly for women.

Grieving is exhausting. In truth, my first few walks were not particularly brisk, but they were as vigorously heart-pumping as I could manage. Start as slowly as you like . . .

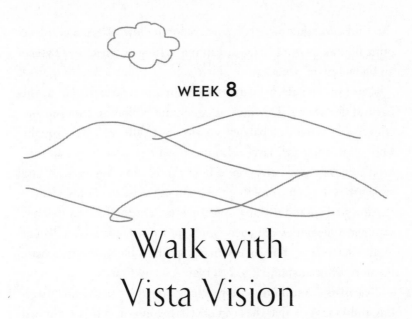

WEEK **8**

Walk with Vista Vision

IN 1987, DR. FRANCINE SHAPIRO was walking in her local park when she noticed that the simple process of scanning the landscape made her feel calmer and less anxious. After years of research, she developed a therapy that mimicked this process but could be used indoors by therapists making a series of hand movements. The therapy—known as EMDR, eye movement desensitization and reprocessing—has been successfully used on thousands of people with PTSD and validated in over fifty studies. But its success is rooted in eye movement, something that happens involuntarily as we stroll. So how does this work?

When we walk in a forward motion, our eyes scan ahead automatically. Dr. Andrew Huberman, a neuroscientist at the Stanford School of Medicine and founder of the Huberman Lab, describes this as "panoramic vision," a way of looking that absorbs the entire scene around us. Panoramic vision is the antithesis of the intense focal vision we use to work on a screen, read a book, or look at our phones. When we engage our eyes in panoramic vision, we absorb the landscape in a process known as optic flow. We can think of optic flow as a sort of visual streaming, telling us where we're going and how best to navigate.

Our eyes contain miniature brain circuits, a layer of cells at the back of the retina that, during panoramic vision and movement, trigger our system of balance so we don't fall over. But, equally important, these cell layers also quiet feelings of anxiety and fear. Studies have shown that optic flow causes our eyes to scan and sweep the landscape, quieting the brain's threat-detection system— the amygdala—and making us feel calmer. During EMDR therapy, traumatic memories are successfully processed not with talk but with a set of eye movements that appear to block the traumatic memory while enabling it to be organized and stored.

Scientists are still unpacking exactly how this works, but emerging studies suggest that the layer of cells behind the retina are linked to our ability to process, store, and retrieve memories from our hippocampus. Huberman's work posits that wide panoramic vision relieves our brain of the close looking and narrow scrutiny that take up so much of our time, but his studies also indicate that a broad-sweeping vision shifts us into a state of greater calm. He speculates that, as hunter-gatherers, our vision and brain developed so that we could navigate and spot water or animals calmly, switching to focal vision (which is inherently more demanding) only when necessary. Today we spend increasing amounts of time focused on close work, depriving our eyes and brains of the panoramas that our nomadic forebears committed to memory. Could this explain why the eye movements that come quite naturally as we walk help us effectively organize difficult memories?

To fully benefit from the therapeutic nature of walking, we need to walk with our eyes. When we're in new locations (on vacation, for instance), our eyes and our brains will be more rigorously engaged, scanning and checking an unfamiliar landscape. Try a new route— visit a cemetery or woodland you've not walked before.

But we can also engage vista vision on our regular local walks by taking the time to look at the full scene and by paying attention to our surroundings. If we unplug from our phones, if we lift our heads, we are more likely to note changes in weather, the turning of the seasons, or a murmuration of starlings, for example. When we walk with our heads tilted and our gaze lifted, we see things we haven't noticed before—architectural details, changes in the tree canopy, bizarre cloud formations, the iridescent flash of a bird's wing. Huberman suggests that despite our greater relaxation, our reaction times are faster when we use panoramic vision.

TIPS

AS YOU WALK, REGULARLY LIFT your gaze from treetops or chimneys to the sky to the horizon.

Try sweeping your gaze horizontally along the skyline—it's thought that a horizontal sweeping motion is particularly effective for inducing a sense of calm.

Pay attention to your peripheral vision—it is often from the corners of our eyes that we spot wildlife (or a sudden car). Our peripheral vision declines as we age, more so if we don't use it, and studies show walking helps restore it.

Want to walk faster? Research suggests that fixing our gaze on something immediately ahead (a tree, for example) causes us to accelerate by 23 percent—and with greater ease—than if we look around.

Borrow one of the many techniques used by writer and walker Nan Shepherd, who—to see the world afresh—would bend over and view it from between her legs, making the landscape "upside down," and exclaiming, "How new it has become!"

Walking backward (see Week 49, p. 202) allows us to engage panoramic vision in an entirely novel way, thereby supporting our brain and our knees.

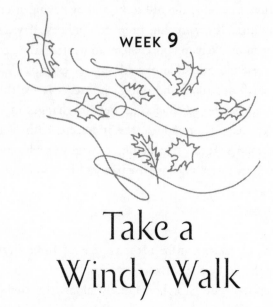

Take a Windy Walk

IN 1911, DOUGLAS MAWSON, AN Australian geologist and explorer, led an expedition to a far-flung pocket of Antarctica. In this dark, ice-cold corner of the world, he and his team perfected the art of *hurricane-walking*—a form of on-foot locomotion that made full use of the endless raging winds. Mawson never forgot the high winds of Antarctica, later writing "a plunge into the writhing storm-whirl stamps upon the senses an indelible impression seldom equaled in the whole gamut of natural experience."

What is it about windy walks that stamp them so indelibly on our memories? People living within the path of famously wild winds (like the Swiss foehn, the French-Spanish tramontana, or the bora, which blasts from Italy through Albania) report deeply polarized experiences. Many love the vigor and freshness of their home wind, like Van Gogh, who attributed his racing, impassioned painting to the intensity of thought triggered by the mistral.

In Eritrea, wind is referred to as *tuum nifas*, meaning a nourishing wind, a breeze that feeds our soul. And in Holland, taking a windy walk is known as *lekker uitwaaien*, which translates as a nice outblowing. For the Dutch, *lekker uitwaaien* is akin to an emotional spring clean: our old dust is pleasantly whooshed away, leaving us invigorated, revitalized, and primed to start over.

But can wind really affect us? Hippocrates certainly thought so, urging caution when winds blew from the north, south, or west. Eastern winds, he claimed, were healthy.

Biometeorology (the study of how atmospheric conditions impact us) is still in its infancy, but when it comes to wind, several theories have been mooted. Does the increase in ozone affect us? What about the fluctuating pressure? Forty years ago, the scientist Lyall Watson hypothesized that ferocious winds induce a typical stress response, pumping adrenaline through our blood and around our bodies: "Metabolism speeds up, blood vessels of the heart and muscles dilate, skin vessels contract, the pupils widen and the hair shows a disturbing tendency to stand on end, producing prickles of apprehension."

Sixty years ago, two Israeli scientists began studying the hot, dry *sharav* wind of North Africa, coming to the conclusion that strong winds affect us physiologically. They speculated that the greater concentration of positive ions in tumultuous winds triggered an overproduction of serotonin. Later studies have been more ambivalent, but it's now recognized that many of us are affected by the weather, with preferences that often run in families, as if our liking or disliking for certain climates is embedded in our DNA.

And while everyone loves a cool breeze on a hot day, vigorous blustery winds are more likely to polarize us—as borne out by a Swedish study that found higher wind speeds improved the mood of some walkers but lowered the mood of others. An earlier study found that women were more responsive to weather conditions—including wind—than men.

The artist Georgia O'Keeffe had a penchant for windy walks, perhaps harking back to her Dutch roots. Her early letters gust with repeated references to thrilling and exhilarating windy walks. "I like the wind—it seems more like me than anything else—I like the way it blows everything . . ." she wrote in 1917. For O'Keeffe, a walk in the wild winds of the Southwest was the perfect energizer, blowing away lassitude and lethargy, and shooing off all seeds of discontent.

O'Keeffe walked the deserts and plains, but breezy forest walks bring their own excitement. In woodlands, we can enjoy the music of wind in trees, particularly white poplars, willows, and pine trees—each of which produces its own song. We hear the rattle of desiccated leaves blowing across the ground, the creaking of trunks, the thrashing of boughs. Lakes too are exhilarating on gusty days— the surface of the water alive with light and movement. On the coast we experience the drama of crashing surf and racing waves. What-ever landscape we choose, a windy walk offers a full sensory experience—we hear, see, and feel it. Much like Mawson's "whirl" that "stamps upon the senses an indelible impression."

Wind also provides a form of natural resistance. As we walk into, or against, the wind, our muscles brace, our leg and chest muscles engage, our lungs work harder. When we walk with the wind behind us, our abdominal muscles are put to work, helping us maintain our balance. For burning calories and building muscles, there's no better walk than an uphill stride in a robust wind!

Wind is an effective disperser of pollution, making windy days (like rainy days) particularly good for urban walks. Both the city and the countryside are also less populated on windy days, not only by people but by mosquitoes and other flying insects that tend to take refuge on gusty days. (Wind also disperses the carbon dioxide we exhale, which is very attractive to mosquitoes, making a windy day a mosquito-free day.) Take advantage and head off for your own refreshing *uitwaaien*.

TIPS

ANYONE CAN ENJOY A WIND walk in a stiff breeze. But if the wind is more akin to Mawson's "writhing storm-whirl," the following will help.

- Tie up long hair, scarves, and loose ends. Wear a hat that hugs the head or straps beneath the chin. Avoid baggy, flapping clothes, and keep pockets zipped.
- If the wind is cold, wear gloves, a windproof parka, and multiple layers.
- Moisturize skin and lips frequently, particularly when the wind is hot and dry.
- Wear sunglasses if the wind is dusty.
- Choose a route protected from the sharper edges of the wind; avoid cliff edges, precipices, exposed areas, and steep ridges.
- Use a clear plastic map protector or GPS on your phone.
- Take hiking poles for additional support and balance.
- Avoid walking in winds above 35 mph, and avoid hilltops, where wind speed will typically be greater.
- Drink plenty of water—wind walking can be dehydrating.
- Want to avoid mosquitoes? You'll need a wind speed equivalent to their flying speed, which is 0.9 to 3.6 mph.

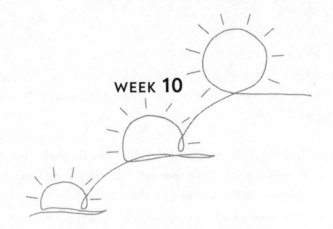

Walk Within an Hour of Waking

"I ALWAYS GO OUT BEFORE it is quite light," wrote the author Harriet Martineau in 1847. "These early walks are good, among other things, in preparing me in mind for my work." Martineau didn't need science to convince her of the panoply of benefits acquired on an early morning stroll. Today, those benefits—those "other things"—have been confirmed. If you take just one daily walk, do it first thing in the morning.

Why? Because light is the primary timekeeper for every cell in our body. And if we get an injection of light *within an hour of waking*, each cell and neuron can set itself accordingly. We don't need hours of light—a ten-minute walk is enough. Nor should we be deterred by poor weather, because even dim and cloudy daylight contains many more lumens (one of the measurements used for light intensity or brightness) than indoor lighting can provide.

Our light sensitivity is at its lowest when we first wake up, meaning we need a bright blast to alert our brain and set our circadian rhythms for the day. Numerous studies have shown that how we spend the first hour of waking can make or break our chances of a good night's sleep. Morning light tells the layer of neurons behind our eyes that it's time to get going, ensuring that our production of melatonin (the hormone that makes us feel drowsy and helps us sleep at night) eases off. But a shock of morning light also sends cortisol flooding through our bodies—waking us up, energizing and invigorating us. Ideally, a few minutes of our morning walk should be without sunglasses, unless it's a dazzlingly bright day.

Morning light also triggers our bodies to make serotonin, a chemical produced by our nerve cells that makes us feel good. Serotonin regulates how well we sleep, later converting to the very melatonin we need to sleep soundly. Odd though it seems, an early morning walk might be the very best thing we can do to improve our nighttime sleep.

Morning light has the potential to do far more than waking us up and helping us sleep. An early morning walk could also protect our hearts: a recent study suggests that bright light can protect and enhance our cardiovascular health by boosting a specific gene that strengthens blood vessels and cuts our risk of a heart attack. Scientists had already spotted a link between light and heart disease, noting the greater prevalence of heart attacks during winter months. But this study revealed something intriguing: participants exposed to thirty minutes of intense light between 8:30 and 9:00 A.M. for five consecutive days had raised levels of a protein called PER2. PER2 is critical for setting circadian rhythms, improving metabolism, and fortifying blood vessels. Earlier versions of the same experiment on *blind* mice found bright light had no effect, hinting at the crucial role our eyes play.

In these experiments, the intense light measured 10,000 lumens.

To put this in context, European daylight ranges from 1,000 to 100,000 lumens depending on time of day and year, latitude and location, and how overcast the sky is. A typical semi-cloudy British morning in winter might reach a peak light intensity of 16,000 lumens. In summer, this rises to around 70,000 lumens. No indoor gym, where the average indoor lumens are closer to 500, can compete. Neither can walking beside a window, because glass filters out some of the UV light that also helps set our biological clock.

It's not only our circadian rhythms that benefit from an early morning walk. A 2012 study found that women who took a brisk 45-minute walk at eight A.M. every day were more active for the rest of the day. They were also less responsive to pictures of food. This was one of the first reports to establish that exercise energizes us while simultaneously—and a little perversely—suppressing our appetite. Some researchers now think we eat less after exercise because brisk movement raises our body temperature, activating hypothalamic neurons that help us control food intake. Just as we eat less when it's warm outside, so we eat less when our bodies are warmed by walking.

But a newer theory posits that we eat less after being active because of a hormone called growth differentiation factor 15 (GDF-15), which our bodies produce when we move. (Two hours of movement can cause our levels of GDF-15 to swell fivefold.) Researchers know that GDF-15 suppresses appetite in rodents and monkeys and are now investigating its effects on human beings. Either way—heat or hormone—an early morning walk may well curb excessive feelings of hunger, helping us regulate and moderate our appetite.

After fourteen years of walking dogs and children every morning, I found myself addicted to a start-of-the-day yomp. Now, like Martineau, I appreciate the opportunity to collect myself, to plan my day: the health benefits are a serendipitous by-product.

TIPS

WALKING BEFORE YOU EAT BREAKFAST has numerous metabolic benefits. See Week 48: Walk Hungry (p. 199).

Still not convinced? Air pollution is often at its lowest first thing in the morning, meaning cleaner air. And in cities, negative ions are most abundant in the morning. Meanwhile, plants release more negative ions into the atmosphere between nine and ten A.M. than at any other time of day, other than eight P.M. For more on ions, go to Week 30: Walk with Ions (p. 122).

Early mornings are the best time to listen out for birdsong: not only are birds more inclined to sing then but, according to the Woodland Trust, birdsong carries twenty times farther than it would later in the day.

Why does birdsong matter? A study from King's College London found that hearing birdsong lifted the spirits of listeners for up to four hours.

Like the sound of boosting your supply of the appetite-suppressing GDF-15? Endurance activities, like tabbing and trekking, are particularly effective. See Week 36: Walk with a Pack (p. 148) and Week 40: Walk Like a Pilgrim (p. 165).

Take a City Smell Walk

ONE MILD FEBRUARY MORNING IN 1790, Jean Noël Hallé, a professor of medicine and Napoleon's private doctor, left his Paris house for a six-mile walk along the banks of the Seine. He took a friend, a map, and his nose. From the Pont Neuf in the center of Paris, the two men walked along the Right Bank, crossing at the Quai de la Rapée, and returning along the left bank. As they walked, Dr. Hallé jotted down every odor. His odor survey was to change the smell of Paris forever, prompting its transition to the fragrant modern city we know today. More importantly, Dr. Hallé was taking history's first recorded smell walk.

Two hundred and twenty years on, Dr. Kate McLean, a designer and cartographer, was walking through Edinburgh sniffing at the air when she noticed the city's distinct smell. It dawned on her that cities carry their own complex, elusive, often fleeting odors. Her epiphany of smell propelled her into a new career as a mapper and artist of smellscapes. In the last decade McLean has guided hun-

dreds of smell walks and mapped the smellscapes of tens of cities—
from Amsterdam to New York to Singapore. As McLean was
walking and plotting smells onto exquisite maps (complete with tiny
bottles of distilled essences reflecting her smellscapes), scientists
were beginning to untangle the complexities of smell, with astonishing results.

Smell is our constant guide, our unsung shadow friend. In the
womb, smell is the only fully formed sense we have. During our first
decade of life, it plays a crucial role in how we experience the world,
our noses able to distinguish billions of different odors. As adults,
we take 24,000 breaths a day, allowing us to savor over 1,000 different smells every hour, via the 5 million smell cells in each of our
nostrils. Except most of us are so busy looking and listening, we pay
scant attention to the heady circulating brew in which we live.

Not so in a few pioneering laboratories where olfaction is being
scrutinized with the scientific rigor it deserves. Some researchers
now think that losing our sense of smell is a more potent predictor
of how long we might live than whether or not we have heart disease. Nor is loss of smell something that affects only older people.
Researchers have linked it to all sorts of conditions, including
depression, schizophrenia, and epilepsy, prompting speculation that
our ability to smell may be considerably more important than previously thought. A study of COVID-19 patients found that loss of
smell and taste were the only coronavirus symptoms linked to
depression and anxiety. Some researchers wonder if losing our ability to smell somehow amplifies feelings of fear and sadness.

How can this be? No one really knows. But when we inhale,
microscopic clusters of scented particles wash over two sets of receptors the size of a thumbprint located at the top of our nostrils. From
here they go to the olfactory bulb in our brain for coding, before
whizzing to the amygdala (the emotional "seat" of our brain) and
the hippocampus (our brain's memory bank) to be filed as a sort of

sensory scented "image." Smell is the only sense that travels so directly, meaning that smell, emotion, and memory are often interwoven and stored as a single file. It's no wonder a simple sniff can spark a vividly evocative memory.

Our ability to smell is much like a muscle: if we don't use it, we risk losing it. But studies suggest that we can often restore our olfactory range. One such study involved twenty people unable to smell a pheromone called androstenone, commonly found in truffles, bacon, and human sweat. Three times a day, for three minutes, participants sniffed away. After six weeks, half of the group could—for the first time—smell the pungent musky aroma familiar to so many of us. Moreover, although our smell cells are replaced every thirty to forty-five days, some participants learned the smell of androstenone in as little as a week.

Smell training does more than improve our ability to identify odors: a striking 2019 study found that after six weeks of smell training, the brain structures of the thirty-five young participants had altered. By using MRI scans, the researchers spotted increased cortical thickness in several brain areas. What does this mean? The cerebral cortex is a tightly folded sheet of neurons wrapped around our brain: think of it as the brain's outermost layer, a sort of snug-fitting coat. The thinning of this layer is often a sign of disease. Much as a threadbare coat can't keep us warm, a threadbare cerebral cortex can't properly preserve our brains. In this instance, cortical thickening took place in brain parts associated with memory and recognition, suggesting that improving our sense of smell may improve our memory too.

I took up smell walking after losing my sense of smell having caught COVID-19. A smell walk with Dr. McLean was a welcome reminder of how *scent* and *odor* add to the sheer joy of being alive. Walking nose to air, pursuing the odorous notes of an English town, we followed a trail of . . . damp leaves, diesel/smell of bus, soil, after-shave, stale clothes, pine tree, wet cardboard, dust, paint, detergent, bleach, smell of hair salon, fresh coffee, sweet warm baking, diesel (again), gutted fish, and pizza.

TIPS

WALK NOSE-FIRST—MCLEAN CALLS THIS scent-catching. Note: it won't work if you have a blocked nose or a hangover.

Drink water. According to Victoria Henshaw (who pioneered the use of smell in town planning), if our noses aren't adequately hydrated, our smell receptors can't decipher odors as well.

Look for variety. Henshaw suggested open *and* enclosed spaces, green *and* concrete spaces, upmarket *and* run-down spaces. The greater the variety, the greater the range of smells.

Use ears and eyes to seek out odor opportunities, from bakeries to florists and from hedgerows to hospitals. Put your nose into shrubs and shops. Always disregard the puzzled stares of passersby!

The smell of a city constantly changes; try the same smell walk in spring and then in autumn, in heat and during rain, at dawn and at night. During night walks (see Week 46: Take a Night Walk, p. 190), we are particularly susceptible to smell.

Our smell receptors tire easily. To rest and reset them, McLean recommends sniffing the skin in the crook of our elbow for a bit.

Take notes if you like. (The language of smell is sparse, so experiment with metaphor—the smell of romance, secrets, home.) Use your notes to create your own smell map or artwork.

We smell less acutely when it's very cold: save smell walks for milder weather.

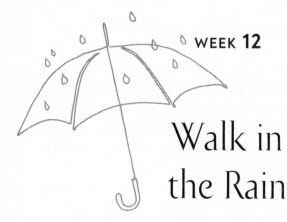

Walk in the Rain

ALTHOUGH MANY OF US SEE a rainy day as a reason for being indoors, a walk in the rain reconnects us with the elements, immediately and directly. As rain stipples our skin, we are—quite literally—touched by nature. Wherever we are, walking in rain is a profoundly physical experience, awakening our sense of touch and reminding us that we are embodied beings.

When rain falls, the increased moisture and the persistent pounding of raindrops cause specific compounds to be released and combined in the air we breathe. It so happens that the simple act of inhaling these compounds can have profound effects on our sense of well-being.

Walking in rain also awakens our sense of smell. Rain releases scents from trees, plants, and soil, imbuing the landscape with startlingly complex fragrances. The Scottish writer and walker Nan Shepherd noted that birch trees after rain release a smell that's "fruity like old brandy," intoxicating enough to leave the walker "as good as drunk." The thrill of fragrance isn't restricted to birch trees. It comes from compounds created and released by a group of oils that plants secrete to prevent them growing too vigorously in periods of dry weather. First noticed on clay (argillaceous) soils, where it's most marked, the soil-after-rain smell was originally spoken of as argillaceous odor, but in 1964, two Australian mineralogists gave a name to this pungent earth-after-rain scent: petrichor. In India, petrichor—which is at its strongest after a period of dryness—has existed as a bottled perfume, known as *mitti attar* or "perfume of the earth," for half a century. We can fill our noses with this extraordinary scent merely by walking in (or directly after) rainfall.

Scientists now think other fragrances are produced by rain as it disturbs and shifts odoriferous molecules from all sorts of surfaces, including the tiny hairs on leaves. While earthy smells are often warm and musky, leaf scent can be clean and astringent—creating a deeply relaxing cocktail of fragrance. Cities aren't immune: rain releases fragrances stored in stone and concrete, although not all are as uplifting as their rural counterparts.

Importantly, rain washes away the vestiges of pollution. Air is always cleaner during and immediately after a downpour. How does this happen? As rain tumbles through the atmosphere, each drop attracts hundreds of pollutant particles, including soot and microscopic particles of PM2.5, leaving the air bracingly fresh, scrubbed clean.

Rain also increases the negative-ion count in the air, which some scientists think might improve cognition, relaxation, and mood. In their book *Your Brain on Nature*, Drs. Eva Selhub and Alan Logan cite several studies suggesting that negative ions (molecules carrying an extra negative charge and found abundantly in forests and moving water) improve health, cognitive performance, and longevity (see Week 30: Walk with Ions, p. 122).

Rain changes everything—touch, sounds, smells—but most of all, it changes what and how we *see*. On a rain-slick walk, tree trunks glitter and gleam, leaves sparkle, petals glisten. Rain makes foliage and flowers translucent so that every vein and marking becomes magically visible. Flowers, boughs, and feathered grasses shift shape, their heads arching and bowing beneath the weight of water. In the rain, a walk we've taken a hundred times becomes a dramatically different experience, jolting our brain to life with a surge of dopamine (see Week 41: Walk to Get Lost, p. 170).

As if this isn't enough, one study also suggests that we burn more calories while taking exercise in the rain. Having tested the participants' blood and exhaled breath, the researchers concluded that: "Minute ventilation, oxygen consumption and levels of plasma lactate and norepinephrine were significantly higher in rain." Put simply, when it's cold and wet, our bodies have to work harder, chomping up calories in the process.

In the rainforests of Uganda, male chimpanzees often dance at the onset of rainstorms, charging through the foliage, beating at the ground, drumming the pink soles of their feet against tree trunks, and flailing at the air with their long arms. No one knows why they rain-dance, but it's a magnificent image, reminding us of the intoxicating possibilities of rain.

TIPS

BUY THE BEST WATERPROOFS YOU can afford, including waterproof pants that tighten at the ankle (to prevent sodden hems leaching water into your boots) and a parka with a peaked hood.

Waterproofs have to be regularly re-waterproofed using a product like Nikwax. Otherwise, they won't stay waterproof, however much they cost!

Ensure you have waterproof walking boots, Wellingtons, or duck boots. Walking boots, like waterproof clothing, need maintaining with dubbing wax on leather, a waterproof spray on nubuck, or a multipurpose waterproof spray for fabric boots.

Urban walking? Consider a fold-away umbrella and/or fold-up waterproof poncho.

Take a Walk-Dance
or a Dance-Walk

IN 1599 A FRIEND OF William Shakespeare called Will Kemp Morris danced 127 miles from London's Royal Exchange to Norwich. It took him nine days, providing him with enough material to write a book. Four hundred years later, a group of Morris dancers repeated Kemp's walk-dance, completing it one day faster. Time after time dance has been proven to lift mood, improve balance, and boost aerobic fitness. So why don't more of us dance as we walk?

As it happens, dancing isn't dissimilar to walking. Many dance moves are more elaborate extensions of walking—the fox-trot, for example. Sadly, most opportunities to dance involve being indoors, often at inconvenient times (like during the night, which is fine if you're a clubber). And predictably, few of us believe we can dance despite being accomplished walkers. Nevertheless, I like to break up my walks with short bursts of dance. I like how it makes me *feel*—the sudden rush of blood and dash of heartbeat as I wave my arms in the air introduces a new element of movement and a shot of joy. Moreover, when the air is bitingly cold, a quick jig or disco dance is an effective way of warming up.

Psychologists have found that simple practices, such as dancing or singing as we walk, help make us "more playful and . . . more satisfied with our lives." Researchers at Germany's Martin Luther University Halle-Wittenberg (MLU) found that a week of playfulness exercises not only improved participants' moods but helped them develop the *trait* of playfulness, potentially leading to more joyful lives. The 533-participant study discovered that inherently playful people (not the same as silly or frivolous) can "turn almost any everyday situation into an entertaining or personally engaging experience." After a week of consciously being more playful, even those who considered themselves serious were better able—and more likely—to incorporate extra play into their lives, leading to "an improvement in . . . well-being." The researchers believe we can all "consciously integrate playfulness into everyday work" (or everyday walk), leading not only to greater life satisfaction but to greater creativity and "more fun."

And yet incorporating play into our lives does more than make us feel good. In 1964, Marian Diamond, one of the founders of modern neuroscience, conducted a groundbreaking experiment on rats in which she proved that rats with access to playthings had larger brains. Subsequent experiments came to the same conclusions, finding "enriched" rodents had greater levels of BDNF (brain-derived neurotrophic factor is vital for growing and preserving brain cells), better memories, and sharper cognition. The message? Play is not just for children.

Dr. Peter Lovatt, psychologist and founder of the Dance Psychology Lab at the University of Hertfordshire, told *The Times* that adding improvised dance into our walking lifts our mood by releasing dopamine (the brain chemical that makes us feel good). It also improves the quality of our thought and decision-making while simultaneously fine-tuning our spatial awareness. He believes that improvising a few dance steps "shakes up our set patterns of behavior," helping us think differently, and turning our walk into a full-blown cognitive workout for the brain. He may be right: a 2012 study found that walkers who moved more fluidly, waving their arms in a sort of improvised dance-walk, generated many more ideas than normal walkers.

TIPS

CHECK YOUTUBE FOR VIDEOS OF how to disco-walk or how to "up-groove" your walk with easy dance steps.

Dance-walk on a smooth surface wearing appropriate footwear.

According to a study from McMaster University, to protect our brain health we should walk briskly for four minutes, followed by three minutes of easy walking—repeated three times. Just swap out the brisk walk for a booty shake, then walk as normal. Repeat.

Dancing can be replaced with skipping or galloping (Miranda Hart style). Both are particularly effective when walking with children, and both increase the aerobic intensity of your walk while simultaneously adding to the play (and feel-good) factor.

Singing as you walk is also surprisingly uplifting (see Week 27: Sing as You Stride, p. 110).

Worried about being seen dancing or singing as you walk? Quiet streets and remote locations offer extra privacy, as do early mornings or evenings, when fewer people are around.

Treasure hunting—either the old-fashioned way or using a scavenger hunt app like Geocaching, Let's Roam, ScavengerHunt.com, or GooseChase—is an easy way to turn an everyday walk into an adventure in play.

Balls are not just for dogs. Throwing a ball as you walk has the additional advantages of improving your balance, stability, coordination, and spatial awareness, while also keeping younger walking companions playfully entertained.

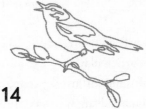

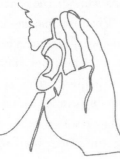

Walk
with
Your Ears

IN JOHANNA SPYRI'S *HEIDI* BOOKS, little Heidi leaves her grand-father's Alpine cabin to live in the city of Frankfurt, where she becomes desperately homesick. Every night she dreams of "the wind in the fir trees." The music of wind shooshing through pine needles runs, like a soundtrack, through Spyri's tale of healing among the mountains.

From the soaring notes of a songbird to the breeze hissing in the leaves, natural sounds have a miraculous power to distract, to con-sole, to soothe. And now researchers are beginning to unpick the reasons for this. Several studies of hospital inpatients have found that listening to natural sounds decreased anxiety, while research into the sound of flowing water found it lowered cortisol levels more effectively than silence or classical music.

Three years ago, a team from Brighton and Sussex Medical School investigated further, measuring the heart rate and brain activity of seventeen healthy young adults as they listened to a variety of natural and artificial soundscapes. The team found that the brain regions typically active when we're resting and relaxed (sometimes called the default mode network) changed according to whether the soundscape was rolling waves or rumbling traffic. When participants listened to rolling waves, their brains switched into what the researchers described as an outward-directed focus of attention. But traffic sounds had a very different effect. Participants' brains switched into an inward-directed focus of attention, remarkably similar to states of mind observed in people with anxiety, trauma, and depression. Think of it as the difference between a mind turning in on itself and a mind reaching out of itself.

It wasn't only the participants' brains that shifted focus as the soundscape changed. Their bodies followed suit. Listening to natural sounds slowed their heart rate, relaxed their muscles, and spurred gentle activity in their intestines and glands, all of which are indicative of the body slipping into a state of active relaxation.

Finally, while listening to natural sounds, the participants performed better in tasks requiring their full attention. In other words, natural sounds were less distracting than artificial sounds, suggesting that tuning into the flow of water as we walk might enhance our problem-solving skills. Interestingly, the researchers found that individuals with the most marked stress were those who relaxed most while listening to natural sounds.

Noise is one of the many stressors in our modern lives. The World Health Organization believes that traffic noise alone accounts for the loss of a million years of healthy life. Numerous reports have exposed the hidden costs of urban noise: a raised risk of hypertension, diabetes, obesity, heart attack, and heart disease. An American study found that noise exposure caused a spike in stress, resulting in inflamed blood vessels, raising the risk of a stroke. Studies of schools near major airports repeatedly find pupils with poorer recognition, memory, and literacy skills, even after adjusting for other variables.

Noise—even the noise we think we've adjusted to—affects our pulse, heart rate, and blood pressure, even in our deepest sleep.

The answer to all this noise is to take a walk somewhere quiet, somewhere we can listen, uninterrupted, to the natural world. According to a study commissioned by the UK's National Trust, the following sounds bring us the greatest pleasure:

- birdsong
- a running stream
- wind rustling tree leaves
- silence
- twigs snapping underfoot
- animal noises
- wind whistling through trees
- rain falling on leaves
- acorns hitting the ground
- squelching mud

This study found that listeners to natural sounds reported a 30 percent increase in feelings of relaxation, while listeners of a guided voice meditation app reported no change in mood. The message is arrestingly clear: turn off your phone, put away your binoculars, and open your ears. People hearing birdsong recorded the highest levels of well-being, with 40 percent saying that birdsong made them feel happy. But don't think listening to an app indoors will have the same effect. It won't. An earlier study found that indoor listeners of recorded natural sounds felt "significantly" less relaxed and energized than those listening to the real thing—outside.

The most effective listening walks require an element of surrender.

Be prepared to let your ears lead, to follow a particular bird or insect, or to explore a more mellifluous section of woodland. The writer Thomas Hardy believed we could recognize tree species by their susurration, the particular sound made by a tree's leaves in the breeze.

Drought, rain, wind, and snow bring new soundscapes, transforming the same old walk into something entirely novel. Night walks (see Weeks 46: Take a Night Walk, p. 190, and 34: Walk Beneath a Full Moon, p. 139) have the same transformative effect, while nocturnal city walks can thrillingly reinvent an urban soundscape. Wherever you choose to walk, following your ears is outward-directed attention at its most focused.

TIPS

LISTENING WALKS ARE BEST DONE alone and in areas of fewer people. Avoid the usual trails, and forget about hunting out a beauty spot—this walk is for your ears rather than your eyes.

Listen out for the more obvious susurrations, like poplar trees, or see if you (like Hardy) can tell one tree from another by the distinctive rustle and rattle of its leaves.

Cup your hands around your ears, or push them forward and away from your head, to amplify the sounds around you.

Close your eyes every now and then to refocus away from the visual and back to the auditory.

Try downloading a recording app and making your own natural soundscape to play as you walk or to send to a friend.

New guided walking apps (like Echoes interactive sound walks) offer novel walking experiences that include historical, geographical, and musical accompaniments. Download and listen for a very different ear-led wander.

Birdsong identification apps are invaluable for learning to differentiate birdcall, one of the great joys of walking with one's ears.

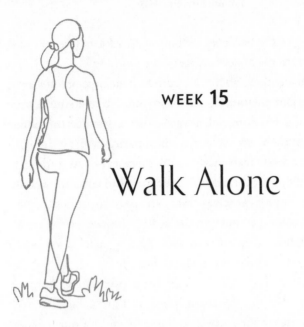

WEEK **15**

Walk Alone

IN 1947, THE AUSTRALIAN-BORN WRITER and market gardener Clara Vyvyan wrote about her frequent and often overwhelming need for a solitary walk: "My lifelong passion was for the open air, the open road and solitary places . . . I was seeking escape from the haunts of man into the sanctuaries of nature." Vyvyan, who walked all over the world, frequently alone, made no bones of the fact that she preferred the company of hills, valleys, and open roads to that of people. Vyvyan had many friends, but it was walking alone that enabled her to recapture a "long-lost intimacy with dark night, dawn . . . wind and the sea." In her walking solitude she forgot herself entirely, hearing only "the pulse of the great world beating."

Vyvyan's perpetual need to walk alone isn't unique. Jean-Jacques Rousseau, William Wordsworth, Henry David Thoreau, Virginia Woolf, Cheryl Strayed, and many others all acknowledged their desire for solitary walks. "A walking tour should be gone upon alone," wrote Robert Louis Stevenson, adding that he had no wish to be restricted by other people. The essayist William Hazlitt thought the very purpose of walking was to be alone, without any "cackle of voices at your elbow to jar on the meditative silence of the morning."

In all the hue and cry about our current pandemic of loneliness, it's easy to overlook the importance of solitude. Recent studies contend that living in our digitized, always-on society makes time alone more important than ever. Solitude—particularly while walking in nature—can be both rejuvenating and therapeutic. According to sociologist Jack Fong, time alone encourages us to confront who we are. When we remove ourselves from our usual social context, we gain perspective. We can nurture the relationship we have with our self. Fong, who takes a monthly solo hiking trip, believes solitude is as restorative and essential as exercise or healthy eating.

Fong's ideas reflect those of the eminent psychiatrist Anthony Storr, who saw the capacity to be alone as a "valuable resource" enabling us to access our deepest feelings. But not in our habitual environment: Storr argued that removing ourselves—as we do when we walk outside—promoted self-understanding and connection with our "inner depths of being," as well as being necessary "if the brain is to function at its best and the individual is to fulfill his highest potential." To support his argument he threw in Buddha, Jesus, and other religious leaders who famously walked alone as a means of self-enlightenment.

Studies carried out in the last couple of years suggest that people able to cultivate solitude are more resilient and more contented. It seems that the greater our capacity for solitude, the less alone we feel. One study found that regular *chosen* solitude resulted in a more positive outlook, less depression, an enhanced ability to manage stress, fewer physical ailments, and greater feelings of satisfaction. Another study suggests that periods of solitude can enhance the quality of our relationships, while a further study finds solitude often stimulates our creativity, bearing out Picasso's saying that "no serious work is possible without great solitude."

A solo hike is a completely different experience from either a group ramble or a walk with a friend, and I urge you to explore it. Walking solo is the ultimate in freedom. We can set off when we like, go where we like, at the time and pace that suits us, for as long—or short—as we like. We can stop when we want, for as long as we want. We can follow any enticing path, valley, trail, alley. Not needing to consult or consider, we are free to do exactly as we please.

And without a companion to help us, we are nudged into self-reliance and, ultimately, self-confidence. The British walker and climber Dorothy Pilley believed her "solitary wanderings with map and compass across the hills" gave her confidence, empowering her as nothing else had. Psychologists refer to this as "self-strengthening."

Alone, we reconnect with nature in a way that is more intense, more meditative, even more meaningful. Pilley found solo walking not only confidence-building but soulfully satisfying:

> To find the top of the Ridge in mist, at dusk, alone and
> come down it, was an adventure that nothing . . .
> would surpass. The curlews wailing over the swamps,
> sheep coughing invisibly out of the grayness on the
> chilly flats, the pinnacles of the ridge looming
> enormous and the wind whistling . . . were impressions
> that stamped themselves deeper than memory.

Recent studies echo this, finding that we are better able to *reflect* and to experience the full splendor of nature when we walk alone.

Incidentally, we often form sharper, more enduring memories when we walk on our own. Psychologists think this is because we have fewer distractions. Instead, we engage more with what's around us, superimposing our memories with greater efficiency and saturation.

Solo hiking is fractionally more hazardous than walking with another person: if we get lost, twist an ankle, encounter a wild animal, or run out of water, there's no one else to rely on. When we walk alone, we need to be fully prepared.

TIPS

SOLITUDE IS HARDER FOR SOME than for others. Start with ten-minute solo walks and build from there.

If you're not (yet) a confident map reader, choose a walk that is navigationally undemanding, like following a river or a canal, or a designated walking trail, or a cliff path.

Leave early in the day, and allow ample time. This reduces any chance of being lost at nightfall.

Take a phone and a spare battery, and let someone know your route and estimated time of return.

Don't carry more than you need—there's no one to share the load.

Take sufficient water and food—there's no one to share their provisions with you.

Walk when the risk of bad weather and/or wild animals is very low.

Nervous about solo walking? Avoid dangerous routes, and consider taking a short navigation course (as I did!).

Concerned about assault? Choose a less empty route (for example Week 17: Follow a River, p. 67), and opt for a weekend, when paths are typically busier. Alternatively, carry a personal alarm, don't wear earbuds, and take heart from the hundreds of female writers and bloggers who hike regularly and safely by themselves.

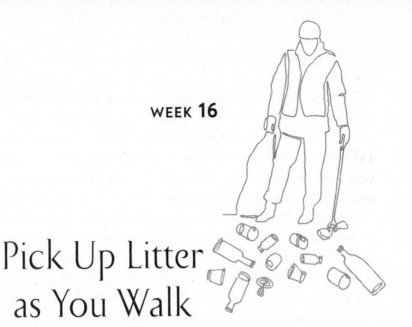

WEEK 16

Pick Up Litter as You Walk

IN THE MIDDLE OF THE COVID-19 pandemic, Danielle Wright, the organizer of a litter-picking group in the English city of Salford, began receiving emotional emails from some of her fellow volunteers. Litter picking, they wrote, had saved their lives, preserved their sanity, and provided them with the social interaction that a national lockdown had deprived them of. "Litter picking helps your mental health . . . it's really rewarding," Wright told her local newspaper.

Throughout the lockdown, Wright's group of litter pickers—who called themselves the Salford Litter Heroes—met daily, sometimes collecting as many as thirty bags of rubbish as they walked, picked, and chatted. The truth about collecting litter is that it provides much more than exercise—a sense of purpose, a chance for social interaction, and the opportunity to leave the landscape in a better state than we found it. Incidentally, litter picking means bending, stretching, and carrying as we walk, turning a litter pick into a full-body workout.

Litter picking invites ready conversation: when I litter-pick with my family, passersby frequently pause to ask what we're doing or simply to thank us. Wright's team—many of whom lived alone—received the same response: discarded rubbish became the spark that kindled conversation, over and over again. When the government restricted outdoor activity to an hour a day, many of Salford's litter pickers chose to spend that hour cleaning the streets of fast-food wrappers, beer cans, and cigarette butts. One of the little unexpected joys of litter picking is the almost instant feeling of pride it engenders. Unlike many activities, litter picking provides immediate visible results. Danielle Wright describes this as "a feel-good feeling . . . good for the environment and good for you."

We know that litter harms wildlife. Animals and birds cut themselves on glass and cans, trap their heads inside jars, become tangled in plastic six-pack rings, suffocate inside plastic bags, ingest toxic waste and latex balloons, get stuck to chewing gum, choke on elastic bands—and so on. The RSPCA receives more than 7,000 calls a year for help with animals hurt or poisoned by litter. Every bit of litter we collect makes a difference. For those of us suffering from eco-anxiety, a litter-picking amble offers an empowering sliver of hope.

The existential power of a litter pick was confirmed when environmental psychologist Dr. Kayleigh Wyles ran a series of beach-walking experiments. Three groups of students were assigned to three different beach-based activities over the course of a week. The first group walked the coastal path, the second investigated rock pools, and the third walked *and* collected litter. While the coast-path walkers reported the greatest feelings of calm, the beach cleaners reported the greatest feelings of meaning and purpose.

Meanwhile, research shows that litter begets litter. People are more inclined to toss their fast-food bag out of a car window if the shoulder they're driving past is already awash with such bags. In this respect, litter picking achieves considerably more than cleaner shoulders and safer wildlife—it has the potential to change human behavior for the better.

Forty years of research have consistently found that volunteering has more therapeutic benefits than we might imagine. People who regularly volunteer have better mental and physical health: less depression, greater self-esteem, lower blood pressure, and reduced rates of mortality.

Recent studies suggest that volunteering keeps our brains sharp. In a 2017 study published by the Oxford University Press, volunteers had better working (short-term) memory and better information-processing abilities than their nonvolunteering counterparts.

Last but not least, our brains reward us for doing good deeds, generously gifting us a shot of dopamine, the feel-good brain chemical that makes us lightly euphoric. Neuroscientists call this "the helper's high," and it can be unleashed by the simplest of things—a passerby thanking us for collecting rubbish, or the sight of a satisfyingly large haul of litter at the end of a pick. Which is merely to confirm that a litter-picking walk makes us feel good in multiple ways while also benefiting wildlife, the environment, and our community. Few walks can claim to achieve quite as much.

TIPS

JOIN A LOCAL LITTER-PICKING GROUP for a chance to socialize as you pick, or go alone, as you prefer.

No local group? Organize one and celebrate your first litter-picking walk with coffee and cake, or a barbecue.

Going alone? Podcasts, an audiobook, or an app like thewalk game.com make excellent companions. Use a single AirPod/earbud so you can hear oncoming traffic.

Wear a high-visibility jacket (or bright clothes) and rubber gloves and/or beg, borrow, or buy a litter picker.

Take two trash bags—one for recyclable litter and one for landfill.

Want to help but can't face litter picking? Use an app like Charity Miles to raise money for good causes as you walk.

Prince Charles famously took William and Harry litter picking as children. And if the royal family can pick up litter . . . enough said.

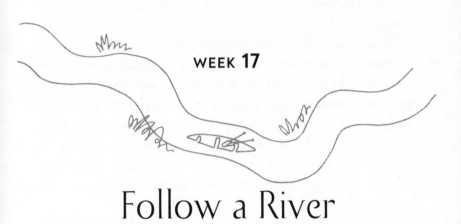

Follow a River

IN 1951, WHEN THE WRITER Clara Vyvyan needed to recover from a series of personal setbacks, she chose to follow a river. "Would I really be able to lose myself in the River Rhone?" she asked. "Lose this wretched, frustrated, disillusioned person that I had become?" As it happened, Vyvyan finished her 462-mile river walk "in a mood of exultation," her happiness fully restored. A river walk doesn't have to be lengthy or wild. On October 30, 1935, the author Anaïs Nin wrote in her diary: "walked along the Seine . . . so happy to be near the river." What is it about following a river that makes us feel so happy?

Although research into blue space (landscapes that include water) has lagged behind studies of green space, our inherent love of water—from lakes to fountains, from oceans to rivers—has been recognized by painters, poets, and garden designers for centuries. The science is finally catching up, helping us understand why we find water both exhilarating and restful, and why the presence of water might genuinely possess curative properties.

Twenty-five years ago, researchers found that a landscape that included running water had a restorative effect on the mood of those passing through it. Was it the sound of water? The light reflecting from its surface? The proximity of potential drink and food (fish)? Or were we simply more physically active when near to water? We still don't fully understand why being close to water makes us feel so good. But today's technologically sophisticated studies use mobile health sensors to capture data on our heart rate, the level of stress biomarkers in our blood, and changes in our brain. And the data is unequivocal: the presence of water makes many of us feel calmer. Water, it appears, may help reverse the stress and overstimulation fostered by our twenty-first-century way of life.

Studies show that women complete longer and more strenuous exercise programs when looking at water, that people spending more time near water report greater feelings of happiness and less depression, and that women listening to the sounds of running water secrete less of the stress hormone cortisol than women listening either to music or silence.

Of course other factors could be at play: the air is less polluted near moving water; the sounds of water blot out aggravating urban noise (see Week 14: Walk with Your Ears, p. 55); we're often *moving* beside water—either walking or doing water sports—which might contribute to our greater sense of well-being; and water is cooling, reducing the discomfort caused by high temperatures.

Proponents of attention restoration theory believe our minds unwind more easily in spaces that provide regularity without monotony—landscapes offering an element of novelty combined with predictability. The predictability (the unchanging flow of a river, for example) allows our brains to relax, while the novelty (ripples, the sudden jump of a fish, the wavering reflections) keeps our minds absorbed and engaged. This perfect pairing of regularity and novelty rejuvenates our weary, overcharged brains, making us feel at once energized and tranquil. As we gaze across the glassy surface of a river, our minds empty in a way that mimics the effects of meditation.

After oceans, rivers top the list of "perfect landscapes for brain restoration," according to Wallace Nichols in his book *Blue Mind*. Each to our own—for me, following a river is my absolute favorite walk, whether it's a short stroll at night or a long-distance hike. River walks require minimal navigation and map reading, making them ideal for either a solo hike or a social saunter where the priority is conversation. This doesn't mean we can switch off altogether. Rivers test our cognitive abilities in unexpected ways (navigating all those meanders, shifting banks, and low-hanging willows), making a river walk equally beneficial for our brains.

Recent studies indicate that we feel more altruistic in the presence of water, as well as experience a greater sense of belonging. Researchers aren't sure why, although I've always found river walks to be particularly social, not only because of the dog walkers, anglers, and cyclists (who like the flat ease of a towpath) but also because of the activity taking place *on* the water—from rowers to houseboats to wild swimmers. Rivers and canals provide both a sense of peaceful tranquility and a feeling of being connected to others, a sense that you're not alone. Nor is it merely the greater number of people we encounter beside a river that makes us feel "accompanied": on a long river walk, the river itself becomes a companion. There's no empirical data to support this, but numerous writers and travelers attest to the strange sense of being *befriended* by a river. I've experienced it myself. In many ways, a river makes not only an incomparable guide but, oddly, the best possible walking mate.

The countryside is crisscrossed by rivers and streams, often rich with wildlife. Identify all those in your vicinity, and plot out routes that work for you. If possible, earmark some longer trails. Start with a full-day hike, then consider a weekend. Two days of river walking requires carrying little more than a change of underwear and a toothbrush. Then try plotting out a longer river walk. Many of the largest rivers now have dedicated walking paths, with places to stay along the way. The Rhône can be walked from source to sea, as can the Thames and Ireland's River Barrow. Many canals and rivers (like Canada's Bow River) have beautiful stretches that can be walked between settlements.

Nor is river walking restricted to the countryside. Cities and towns are invariably threaded by a river or canal, often rich with history, like the celebrated River Walk in San Antonio, Texas.

If you can bear it, include a river dip. Surprisingly, a quick plunge in cold water adds to our feelings of happiness. The chill activates temperature receptors under the skin that trigger the release of adrenaline and feel-good endorphins. Researchers in Bangalore found an hour's immersion increased dopamine levels by 250 percent. In October 2020 the BBC reported on the world's first study of cold-water swimmers, each of whom carried—in their blood—a "cold-shock protein" known to delay the onset of dementia.

TIPS

RIVERS CAN BE DECEPTIVE, WITH lengthy meanders meaning long spates of walking without covering much distance. Use a map or an app.

Microfiber towels are useful after a quick paddle or swim. Always check pollution levels before you swim by looking at local state park websites or contacting the National Park Service.

Take binoculars—rivers are home to plentiful wildlife—and sunglasses to protect against river glare on bright days.

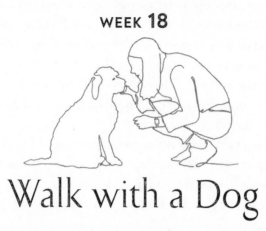

Walk with a Dog

IN **1863, A YORKSHIRE WOMAN** called Mary Eyre did something few Victorian women would have countenanced. She walked alone through the remote Pyrenees, crossing from France to Spain on a network of old mountain tracks, carrying nothing but a small water-proof bag. A journey on foot like this was supremely dangerous for an unaccompanied woman. But Mary felt no fear because she had a companion—a small Scottish terrier that she described as "my guard in my long solitary walks."

Walking with—and without—a dog are very different experi-ences. For fourteen years I walked twice a day with an exuberant black Labrador, instilling in me habits that lived on long after she died. For a few months, walking without her at my side felt immensely sad and slightly odd. Why was I still leaping out of bed at dawn and walking so zealously if I had no dog to trot? I decided it was her legacy to me—my dog had given me the gift of everyday walking, and I would treasure it for as long as possible.

Of course, not all dog walking is the same. Walking a boisterous puppy is nothing like walking a very old dog, and walking a Chihuahua is nothing like walking a border collie. To boot, walking unencumbered is quite different from walking with a dog at your heel or a puppy sprinting into oncoming traffic. But one thing is certain: dog owners (*companions* is a better word, but I'll stick with *owners* for clarity) typically walk more frequently—and for longer—than those without dogs. Researchers call this "the Lassie effect," and studies suggest that the stronger the bond between dog and owner, the more they walk together.

Today there are numerous schemes for those of us who want to walk a dog but don't necessarily want to own one, from local dog-share schemes like borrowmydoggy.com to volunteering at a local dog shelter or rescue trust. No one should adopt a dog in order to walk more.

A 2006 study carried out in Australia and Germany found that people who became long-term pet owners paid considerably fewer visits to the doctor and appeared to be in better health. This could be a result of the additional physical activity proven to accompany dog ownership. For instance, we know that dog owners move for an extra thirty minutes every single day. But dog owners also have to lift, stretch, and bend more than the rest of us, as anyone who has fed and watered a dog will know.

Unsurprising, then, that a Swedish study of over 3 million adults found that owning a dog meant a lower risk of death from any cause, a figure that fell still further if the dog owner lived alone (other than their dog), hinting at the mysterious role played by companionship when it comes to our health. People living alone are normally at higher risk of death than those in multi-person households—but not if they share their lives with a dog. Dog owners also have lower cholesterol levels and lower blood pressure than their non-dog-owning counterparts—perhaps a result of their extra walking.

It's not just our physical health that improves with a dog in our lives. Stroking a dog is known to raise levels of oxytocin (the so-called love hormone) and to cut levels of cortisol (the so-called stress hormone). An experiment among hospitalized children found that access to therapy dogs reduced stress and anxiety. Another study found that older people recovering from strokes relearned to walk more effectively if a rehabilitation dog was involved.

And—as if all this wasn't enough—studies of our microbiomes suggest those of us spending time with dogs have more diverse bacteria in our guts, possibly giving us improved immunity (perhaps another reason that German and Australian dog owners were less likely to visit their doctors). As one American newspaper recently quipped: "Are pets the new probiotic?"

To top it all, older dog owners also appear to enjoy better brain health. How can this be? In his book *The Changing Mind: A Neuro-scientist's Guide to Ageing Well*, Daniel Levitin explains that hiking is essential for keeping our brains youthful. When we hike, he says, we repeatedly encounter situations that require some form of cognitive navigation—branches that must be ducked, rocks and mud that must be avoided, wildlife we don't want to disturb, roads that must be crossed. We also have to make "hundreds of micro-adjustments," he adds, endless tiny decisions about how lightly to land, whether to angle ourselves for better balance, and so on. All of this keeps our brain working, preserving it in the process. Anyone who has walked with a dog knows that geonavigational decisions and micro-adjustments increase when we also have to predict and negotiate the responses of a pooch. When we walk with dogs, we make decisions not only for ourselves, but for them.

The better brains of dog owners might also be a result of the social aspect of dog walking, which often involves conversing with other dog walkers. Perhaps this sheds light on a slightly inexplicable recent finding: that dog owners have higher self-esteem. Could it be that having responsibility for a dog gives us a greater sense of purpose, resulting in amplified feelings of self-worth? Meanwhile, children from dog-owning families have fewer problems getting along with their peers, suggesting a dog may play a role in helping children's social-emotional development.

When I look back (as I often do) on my many years of walking beside a much-loved dog, what I most vividly recall is her rapture at being outside, her constant sniffing curiosity, her sheer delight in moving—racing, bounding, trotting, and in her last months, lumbering, but with as much pleasure as ever. She infected me with the same enthusiasm, helping pull me entirely into the moment. In many ways, my dog taught me to walk, rather than the other way round.

Not all of us have the space, leisure time, or income to home a dog. Besides, walking without a dog brings many of its own pleasures: we can scramble over stiles, walk fret-free through fields of sheep, glimpse more abundant wildlife, and hike without having to pick up dog poop.

But would Mary Eyre have walked over the Pyrenees without her little dog—her *guard* and companion? Somehow I doubt it.

TIPS

BORROW A DOG—FROM A FRIEND, relative, or dog-share scheme—before you commit. You might also try fostering a dog from a local shelter.

Check new routes beforehand: not every walk is dog-friendly.

To get the full postural benefits of swinging both arms (see Week 2: Improve Your Gait, p. 10), make sure your dog has off-lead time.

Dog poop is harmful for the environment and dangerous for some wildlife. Always take it home with you or dispose of it in marked dog-waste bins.

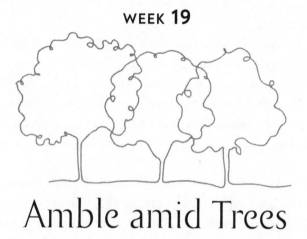

Amble amid Trees

IN 1960, SUNBATHING SCIENTISTS THUMBING through their favorite magazine were dramatically jolted from their beachside reveries. The August issue of *Nature* contained a paper titled "Blue Hazes in the Atmosphere," written by a little-known Dutch biologist called Frits Warmolt Went. The languid title belied its radical contents. Went postulated that the haze we see over the landscape is nothing less than a vast cloud of molecules and gases produced by trees and plants. As light hits the molecules, it scatters—a process known as Rayleigh scattering—leaving the blue, brown, and white haze much loved by fifteenth-century landscape painters.

A Russian biochemist called Boris Tokin had already identified the compounds produced by plants to protect themselves, coining the term *phytoncides*. But it was Frits Went who first grasped the sheer scale of these emissions, not to mention their impact on the earth's atmosphere. Went was decades ahead of his time. His work languished until new technology allowed scientists to measure and analyze these hugely complicated compounds. We are only just beginning to understand their astounding potential, begging the question—can the emissions of trees explain why we feel better after walking in woodland?

We not only *feel* better, we may *be* better. When researchers at the University of East Anglia studied data from 140 reports involving over 290 million people across twenty countries, they found that time spent amid natural greenery had significant and wide-ranging health benefits, including a reduced risk of type 2 diabetes, cardiovascular disease, premature death, high blood pressure, and stress.

Today the spotlight is on woodland. A Finnish study found that adults ("particularly healthy middle-aged women") experienced immediate improvements in well-being after walking among trees. Participants returning from a woodland stroll showed significantly dropped cortisol levels (a marker of stress), reflecting a review of twenty-two clinical studies, which also identified dramatically lower cortisol in the saliva of woodland walkers.

This is old hat in Japan, where researchers have been reporting similar results for two decades. The Japanese, who call it *shinrin-yoku*, or forest bathing, were the first to discover that walking in woodland lowered blood pressure, heart rate, and stress levels, as well as reducing inflammation and improving immunity.

It's not only our bodies that benefit. At Barcelona's Institute for Global Health, researchers found people living in leafy neighborhoods remained mentally sharper. In the UK a similar picture emerged after researchers tested the brains of 6,500 people over ten years, correlating their results with satellite images showing the prevalence of greenery in their respective neighborhoods. Those living with abundant trees and foliage had slower cognitive decline. But it's not only about where we live. When a study of 50,000 teenage pupils found that those *educated* near trees achieved better grades regardless of where they lived, it became apparent that scientists had barely scratched the surface of what makes a tree so therapeutic.

The billion-dollar question, then: Why do trees have such powerful physiological and psychological effects on us? A handful of scientists have nailed their colors to the mast, claiming it's the terpenes, one of the more potent phytoncides produced in the leaves, stems, roots, and trunks of plants.

Most terpene research has been carried out in petri dishes or on rodents. But early results are both promising and exciting. Many terpenes act as powerful anti-inflammatories, including alpha-pinene (found in coniferous trees and rosemary), gamma-terpinene (found in eucalyptus and paperbark trees), and delta-limonene (found in mint, horse chestnut, eucalyptus, juniper, and black walnut). Delta-limonene has also proven to reduce glucose and insulin levels in elderly people, and to be more effective than antidepressants for improving the mood of those with depression.

Anti-inflammatory effects have also been discovered in sabinene, the most abundantly produced terpene in beech trees. Linalool—found in lavender and birch trees—has had excellent results reducing lung inflammation in mice. Several terpenes appear to have anticancer effects (see Walk 39: Walk with Your Nose, p. 161), particularly those found in pine trees. Other terpenes are powerfully antioxidant, like camphene, found in the liquidambar tree. Several terpenes appear to be neuroprotective, like humulene, from the balsam fir tree.

Time in woodland also improves our microbiota. Doctors have long known that children growing up in the wild have richer, more diverse microbiomes, but in 2019 Finnish scientists put this to the test. Tracts of forest floor—including trees and undergrowth—were planted in the playgrounds of city day-care centers. The children were allowed to play for 1.5 hours a day, five days a week. The researchers tested the children's gut and skin for microbes, comparing them to the gut and skin of children in regular day-care centers.

Within four weeks, the microbes of children playing among trees had grown in diversity. In particular, the researchers found plentiful microbes from the gammaproteobacteria family on the children's skin, a strain thought to be vital for our immunity. Intriguingly, the changes in the children's microbiome and skin were reflected by "parallel changes in their immune systems." The more they were exposed to woodland, the stronger their immune systems became.

But let's not be blinded by science. Forests don't exist to serve our health: they are magical places of extraordinary vernal beauty, home to wondrous wildlife and mind-boggling underground skeins of fungi, all of it existing in an intricate and miraculous ecosystem of its own. Tread lightly, move quietly, feel the rush of scented air on your skin, and smell the perfume of terpenes in your nostrils. Few places are as enchanting as a woodland at dawn or dusk . . .

TIPS

DECIDUOUS WOODS HAVE GREATER SEASONAL interest than evergreen: bare branches open up new vistas in winter, while blazing color transforms a forest in autumn.

Touching organic landscaping materials has been shown to immediately increase the diversity of proteobacteria, including gammaproteobacteria, on skin, so take your gloves off and make a point of using your hands.

Evergreen trees provide a greater abundance of terpenes: for the full effect, inhale deeply as you walk. Try brushing past trees or scrunching the odd leaf from different trees (oak, beech, birch, walnut) and smelling their odors to create a sort of woodland smell walk.

Different woodlands produce different blends and quantities of terpenes, so vary your woodland walks and visit at different times of the day and year.

Studies suggest that a two-hour walk is sufficient to significantly increase our natural killer (NK) cells (the cells in our immune system that attack viruses and tumor cells). Meanwhile, three days in woodland increased NK cells by 50 percent in a study carried out by *shinrin-yoku* pioneer Dr. Qing Li.

Take a weekly forest walk if possible. According to a meta-analysis published in the *American Journal of Lifestyle Medicine*, the effects of being in woodland endure for a week.

Help increase woodlands by planting your own trees or contributing to local woodland charities. You can offset your carbon emissions by purchasing trees through schemes like Forest Carbon (forestcarbon.co.uk) or myclimate (myclimate.org).

Seek out arboretums (and pinetums), which often include numerous tree species.

Trees and woodlands become more fascinating with a little knowledge. Invest in some of the latest books on the science of woodlands to have your mind fully blown (see Recommended Reading, p. 257), and download wildlife apps to help identify flora and fauna.

Walk to Remember

A DECADE AGO, PSYCHOLOGISTS IN Germany and the United States began mulling the possibility that walking might be more conducive to memory than sitting in front of a book, screen, or set of flash cards.

The German psychologists found that both children and adults had better working memory (the ability to recall newly learned facts) while walking than while sitting, with the results more marked among children. Recall improved still further when participants set their own walking speed. The researchers didn't have an explanation, but at the same time a similar experiment was taking place in the United States. Psychologists from California State University at Long Beach and the University of Illinois recruited eighty students and asked them to study lengthy lists of nouns. Some of the students took a ten-minute walk before they began studying; some took a ten-minute walk after studying but before being tested; others sat quietly looking at pictures of landscapes before both studying and testing. One group of students far surpassed the others, recalling 25 percent more of the studied nouns. To the researchers' surprise it was the group that took a ten-minute walk *before* they began studying. Walking before being tested made little difference, and the psychologists concluded that taking a ten-minute walk before studying provides "a memory advantage." And yet they still couldn't explain why this happened.

In the intervening decade, our understanding of memory and movement has increased exponentially. After an invigorating walk, we often feel a greater sense of physical and psychological well-being, a feeling that some scientists now attribute to endocannabinoids—tiny molecules produced by our bodies when we do something physically demanding. These molecules circulate through our blood, crossing the blood-brain barrier and binding to cellular receptors in a way still not fully understood. Early studies of our hugely complex, cell-signaling endocannabinoid system have linked it to our ability to sleep, feel happy, reproduce, form muscle, and rebuild bone, among other things. However, recent studies have also linked our endocannabinoid system to our ability to remember, because these microscopic molecules also bind to receptors in the hippocampus—the part of the brain responsible for processing and storing memories. When we walk briskly, our levels of the endocannabinoid anandamide (AEA) increase: some neuroscientists now think that AEA promotes plasticity in our brains, effectively enabling our brains to rewire themselves. Recent studies have sought to link this to our walking speed, posing the question—does our memory improve if we walk more or less quickly?

The answer is . . . both. Different walking speeds trigger different types of memory. A team of Swiss neuroscientists found that thirty minutes of moderate exercise (the equivalent of a brisk walk on flat land) improved associative memory, while very vigorous walking (the equivalent of speed walking uphill) for fifteen minutes dramatically increased levels of endocannabinoids, resulting in significantly improved recall.

Other studies have found that as little as ten minutes of slow walking—the equivalent of an after-dinner stroll—can make a difference, improving communication between various memory pathways. Meanwhile, a new study from Sweden claims that even two minutes of walking has a positive effect on learning and memory in young adults.

Confusing? Not necessarily . . . if you're studying for exams where simple recall is required, factor in periods of power or uphill walking. If you need to use associative memory (linking ideas to names and faces, for example), include periods of brisk walking. Best of all, walk at varying speeds, and for anything upward of two minutes. Ideally, walk at different points while you study—before starting, in the middle (or every hour), and after finishing. On each occasion, and at each speed, different parts of your memory will be activated.

It's not only the timing and speed of our walking that helps us lay down and organize memories. The *direction* in which we walk also has an effect. While many studies have linked motion and memory, one researcher went further. Dr. Aleksandar Aksentijevic, a psychologist at London's University of Roehampton, recruited 114 people to take part in six different memory experiments. After being shown a video of a staged crime, a word list, or a group of images, participants then walked backward and forward or remained sedentary before being quizzed on what they had seen.

In every case, people involved in reverse motion were better able to recall information and past events than those sitting still. In five of the six experiments, memory sharpened when people moved backward. On average, the memory boost lasted for ten minutes after people stopped moving. Dr. Aksentijevic refers to the effect of motion-induced mental time travel as the mnemonic time travel effect.

We know the practical reasons for maintaining a razor-sharp memory, but studies have since revealed a far less obvious motivator. Researchers have discovered that people able to draw from a bank of uplifting memories are more resilient to stress. Being able to recall positive experiences and savor good memories, say researchers, helps us respond to stressful situations with greater emotional resilience. We don't know if walking helps us hang on to old memories in the same way that it helps us recall recently learned facts, but neuroscientists agree that walking prevents memory shrinkage: a 2010 study showed that the keenest walkers (those doing over a mile a day) went on to have the most robust memories in later life, cutting their risk of memory loss in half.

Meanwhile, a 2021 study of people (aged fifty-five plus) already suffering from memory loss found that a walking program improved some of their thinking abilities, prompting speculation that regular movement can slow the path of Alzheimer's.

TIPS

STUDYING FOR EXAMS? MAKE REGULAR walks a part of your timetable, even if it's a gentle two-minute walk between subjects.

Better still, mix up the speed of your walk.

A study published in *Brain Research* found a short burst of movement, like a fast walk, resulted in an improvement in concentration that lasted for an hour. So consider working in hour-long chunks punctuated with short, speedy walks.

Try walking in reverse if you're having trouble recalling.

Don't be tempted into excessively vigorous exercise: a 2017 study found that acute exercise, even in short bursts, led to "a decrease in verbal memory, immediate recall memory, and delayed recall memory," probably because of the subsequent fatigue. Walking is the perfect intensity!

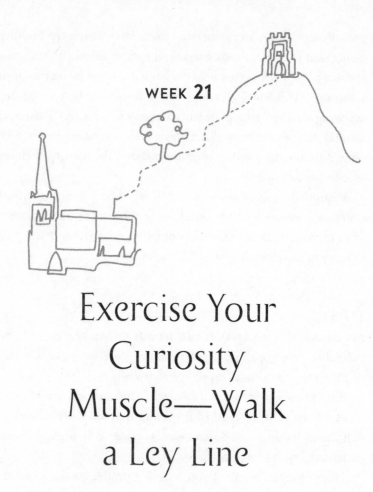

Exercise Your Curiosity Muscle—Walk a Ley Line

ONE WARM AFTERNOON IN THE summer of 1921, Alfred Watkins stood on a hilltop in the English county of Herefordshire admiring the view. It was a landscape he knew well: not only had he lived and worked here all his life, but he was a talented landscape photographer, a keen amateur archaeologist, and an enthusiastic naturalist. And yet that day Watkins (a famously curious man) saw something for the first time, something he'd never previously noticed. He turned from the vista to his map, where he observed an unacknowledged straight line connecting his hilltop to a slew of ancient sites—as if strung upon a straight thread, one after another. It was an epiphany, a "rush of revelations" that changed the course of his life. Watkins raced home and began stabbing steel pins into "sighting points" on maps, drawing straight lines with "astounding results." He maintained that historically salient points—which ranged from castles and churches to mountain passes and standing stones—existed along single straight lines, developed millennia ago as trading or religious routes.

Watkins coined the term *ley lines* to describe this pattern of alignments and argued that a minimum of four salient landmarks constituted a ley line. Although he initially identified them on maps, when he subsequently traveled a ley line, he often found other "sighting points," from streams and springs to fragments of old causeway—all indicative, he believed, of an ancient superhighway walked by our distant ancestors. His ideas—fleshed out and published in two books—courted controversy from the beginning. But the real controversy came three decades after his death, when 1960s New Agers reimagined ley lines not as primitive walking tracks but as secret networks of energy, lines of earth power, cosmic mysteries known to our prehistoric ancestors but lost to us. For many this was a step too far, and Watkins and his theory of ley lines were ridiculed and maligned.

There is no scientific evidence of ley lines. But recent writers have noted that Watkins's ley lines often coincide with medieval pilgrim routes, the paths of underground streams, or long-gone funeral paths. Whether ley lines follow coffin routes, magnetic lines of energy, trading or pilgrim tracks, or none of these is largely irrelevant. To tread a ley line is to walk with curiosity. To plot and follow a ley line exercises our curiosity muscle, raising question after question, inviting us to decode the history and spirit of a landscape, to seek out connections between buildings, geology, geography, place names, plant life, hidden streams, and long-lost trails.

In the last few years the subject of curiosity has been studied by neuroscientists with illuminating results. When Matthias Gruber, principal investigator of Cardiff University's Motivation and Memory Lab, carried out an experiment to examine the links between curiosity, learning, and memory, he found that people made curious by one subject were better able to learn and remember less interesting subjects that came afterward. Brain scans showed that the initial curiosity spurred activity in the hippocampus, which then continued firing long afterward, helping process later—and less interesting— information and memories. "Curiosity affects memory," explained Gruber, putting "the brain in a state that allows it to learn and retain any kind of information."

Earlier studies have linked greater levels of curiosity with greater personal fulfillment, including—oddly—a sort of twenty-four-hour time lag, so that a spike of curiosity results in a sense of "meaning and life-satisfaction" that lingers for a further day. According to professor of psychology Todd Kashdan, curiosity is "one of the most reliable and overlooked keys to happiness," enabling us to experience discovery, joy, and delight. Kashdan's own research also shows that being curious helps us accommodate stress in our lives, beefing up our emotional resilience. Psychologist Edith Eger credits her Auschwitz survival to her curiosity, explaining, "It's what kept me alive . . . I always wanted to know what was going to happen next."

Curiosity also appears to be physically protective. A 1996 study of 1,000 adults found that the most curious lived longer, regardless of whether they smoked or had any sort of disease. Another study discovered that people with greater amounts of curiosity were less likely to develop high blood pressure or diabetes. It's not just our health and happiness that benefit from a strong sense of curiosity: apparently—and perhaps unsurprisingly—curious people also have more satisfying relationships and marriages.

So, suspend any disbelief and all judgment—an open mind is a prerequisite to curiosity—and tap into your inherent inquisitiveness by plotting and walking a ley line.

TIPS

BEGIN BY USING WATKINS'S TECHNIQUE and marking a meaningful point, either man-made or natural, on an official government map. (You need as detailed a map as possible.) Use a ruler or other straightedge to make a line between your first point and other meaningful points. A minimum of four points transforms your arbitrary line into a ley line.

Walk the line, noting any unmapped salient points along the way.

Pay close attention: apparently psychics feel the magnetic energy pulsing beneath their feet on a ley line.

To follow lines already devised by ley hunters, investigate books, websites, blogs, YouTube videos, and ley-hunting groups.

Photography (particularly aerial) can help identify intriguing spots, shapes, or lines that may not be visible to the earthbound eye.

Some ley hunters attempt to align their "significant points" with global landmarks (the Great Wall of China, the Egyptian pyramids, Machu Picchu), making for an engaging geography lesson.

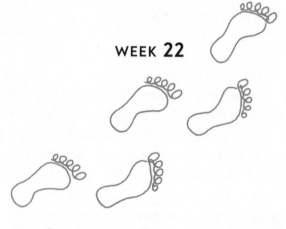

Take a Silent Stroll

A DECADE AGO SCIENTISTS DISCOVERED that rats exposed to loud noise stopped making new neurons in their hippocampi, the brain region linked to memory and learning. In a separate experiment, another clutch of scientists discovered that mice given two hours of silence each day produced new neurons in their hippocampi. The very simple conclusion (noise = bad, silence = good, for the brain at any rate) shouldn't have come as a surprise. As far back as 1859, Florence Nightingale wrote in *Notes on Nursing* that "unnecessary noise is the most cruel absence of care that can be inflicted on sick or well." History is proving her right. Meanwhile, rodents have been replaced by human beings in the latest studies of noise and silence—with startling and unexpected results.

Swedish researchers found that people exposed to traffic noise were more likely to be obese—while those exposed to traffic, railway, *and* aircraft noise were at "a particularly high risk." A study of

380,000 Canadians uncovered a clear link between traffic noise and diabetes, while an investigation of schools found that pupils educated beneath the Heathrow flight path had poorer memory and poorer reading comprehension. A report from the University of Michigan found people living in noisier environments had a 36 percent greater chance of getting Alzheimer's.

Exposure to noise has also been linked to sleep disturbance, heart disease, diabetes, hearing loss, high blood pressure, and stress. Ultimately, prolonged or loud noise leads to hearing loss. When noise damages the minuscule hairs located in our inner ear, our ability to hear is destroyed forever.

Professor Stephen Stansfeld, a world-leading noise expert, argues that even noise we've adjusted to (and no longer hear) affects us—stealing into our ears, vibrating the tiny bones there; morphing into electrical signals that pass to our brain; triggering our stress hormones; disrupting our pulse, heart rate, and blood pressure; upsetting our circadian rhythms. Even as we sleep. Stanfield's advice is to go somewhere deeply and satisfyingly silent whenever we can.

The good news is that silence is as restorative as noise is debilitating. In studies of hospital patients, silence reduced perceptions of pain more effectively than listening to jazz music. A 2006 study on the physiological effects of music—intended to examine how people responded to different musical genres—found that it was not music but silence that had the most dramatic effect on participants' stress markers. Silence was more relaxing than soothing music. Moreover, if the silence came after a piece of music, it was still more relaxing. In other words, silence was intensified by contrast. A later study from the University of Oregon confirmed that the sound-processing bit of the brain doesn't simply pause when noise ceases. Instead, it *responds* to the silence.

When we have nothing to listen to and no sounds to disturb us, our bodies can rest and our brains can get to work building new neurons, a process known as neurogenesis. As such, silence works in much the same way as meditation (which has also been found to trigger the creation of new neurons; see Week 51: Walking as Meditation, p. 211).

But silent strolling, unlike a walking meditation, doesn't mean we have to walk alone. When we walk silently alongside another person, something uncanny takes place. If we like our walking companion (or even if we think we *might* like them in the future), we fall into step with them, an event known as step synchronization. A Japanese study found that less than ten minutes of silent walking with a stranger created a connection or bond, expressed by walkers falling into step and moving with the same speed, stride, and rhythm. In this experiment, participants—unknown to each other—were paired up and told to walk side by side along a quiet path. A motion sensor disguised as a GPS device tracked the synchrony of their footsteps. Paired walkers with more favorable first impressions of each other quickly fell into the same rhythm. After walking a quarter of a mile in silence, their impressions of each other rose still further, indicating that some form of nonverbal communication was taking place. The researchers were surprised to find "first impressions reflected in the subtle action of walking," noting how walking side by side, in silence, favorably altered the relationship between two strangers.

Of course, there is never complete silence. Even in the quietest of places we can hear our breath, our footfalls. But noiseless places exist, landscapes without leaf blowers, traffic, trimmers, car alarms, and airplanes. Seek them out. Unplug from your phone. Observe how silence changes not only the *sound* of things but the *look* of things. In the Himalayas, writer Peter Matthiessen noticed how the light was intensified by the lack of noise.

TIPS

WHEN IT COMES TO RESETTING ourselves, we don't necessarily need a lengthy hike. In the 2006 study quoted above, it took a mere two minutes of silence for the participants' bodies to relax. A two-minute silent phone-free walk in a quiet location may be sufficient.

Resist the need to chat. Walking silently with a companion creates an intimacy as strong as any conversation.

Every now and then stop walking, close your eyes, and simply . . . listen . . .

Try walking as quietly as you can. The additional effort often intensifies our awareness of sound.

WEEK **23**

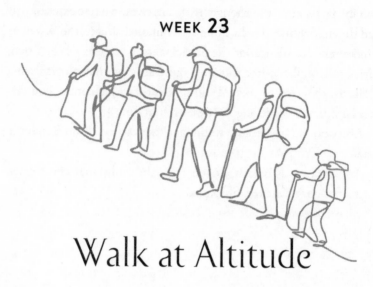

Walk at Altitude

IN THE 1930S A GROUP of Russian scientists began investigating the effects of oxygen deprivation on the human body, a condition known as hypoxia. For decades, hidden away behind the Iron Curtain, the Soviet researchers experimented on both humans and animals. Many of these experiments and trials took place at high-altitude mountain camps. Others took place in altitude chambers, on airplanes, or in laboratories. The researchers examined the effects of both continuous oxygen depletion and intermittent oxygen depletion, quickly realizing that—although the human body cannot survive without adequate oxygen—their experiments were having remarkable results. Eventually they fine-tuned a technique and named it interval hypoxic training (IHT). IHT involved several minutes of exposure to hypoxia followed by several minutes of recovery. It was used to help athletes, asthmatics, and cancer patients, among others.

Sixty years after the Russian experiments started, studies of interval hypoxic training began appearing in below-the-radar Russian medical journals, although all details of the earliest experiments had disappeared without a trace. Curious scientists in the West got wind of the Soviet studies, translated them, and began conducting their own trials. A consensus was emerging: moderate altitude (and mild or intermittent hypoxia) seemed to create biochemical changes beneficial to the human body.

American researchers investigating the links between altitude and chronic disease found people living above 5,000 feet typically lived three years longer than those residing at sea level. The researchers dug a little deeper and found that men and—particularly— women living at altitude were less likely to be obese and far less likely to die from heart disease than their sea-level peers. The same link between obesity, heart health, and altitude was found in Nepal, India, and Argentina. Again and again, people living at altitude appeared to have better health.

At altitude, air is thinner, with fewer oxygen molecules. Our bodies compensate for the reduced oxygen by producing more red blood cells but also by growing new blood vessels that can act as backup routes to the heart. But it's not only our hearts that fare better at moderate altitude. Some cancers and strokes also seem to be less frequent among those living at high elevations. Studies now suggest that thinner air might suppress appetite and increase metabolism, as well as improve immunity, mood, osteoarthritis, and gastrointestinal disease. According to Robert Roach, director of the Altitude Research Center at the University of Colorado Anschutz Medical Campus, fat-burning efficiency improves at altitude, we can think more clearly, and exercise endurance improves. Altitude isn't generally good for people with respiratory disorders, although the Russian scientists had some success treating asthma and chronic lung disease with IHT, and very recent research suggests that some conditions (like chronic obstructive pulmonary disease, one of the world's leading causes of death) are less prevalent at higher altitude.

Fledgling theories abound, but some researchers think the depleted oxygen (which causes the potentially fatal condition hypoxia, when not enough oxygen reaches our cells and tissues) forces the nervous system to fight back, protecting and repairing our cells and neurons in the process.

No one is quite sure how this happens, but elite athletes aren't waiting to find out. Many now train at altitude in order to improve strength, speed, and general performance—and to boost their red blood cells in readiness for races at sea level. In the meantime, a new generation of scientists is busy researching the possibilities of therapeutic intermittent hypoxia for disorders as wide-ranging as spinal-cord injury, multiple sclerosis, and stroke.

Hiking at a moderate elevation is an excellent way to experience some of the benefits of being at altitude. Every year I spend a week walking in the mountains, usually at an altitude between 6,500 and 10,000 feet, mostly because I love the landscape, but also because I find the air energizing and I like the idea that I might be recharging my cells and neurons—somehow. Incidentally, researchers agree that an altitude between 6,500 and 10,000 feet is optimal for enhancing fitness and avoiding the physiological stress of being at very high altitude.

TIPS

DON'T START TOO AMBITIOUSLY, GIVE yourself time to acclimatize, and make your base at a lower level than you intend to walk.

Make sure you're in good shape before you go. If you haven't walked at altitude before and have any medical conditions, talk to your physician. Each of us responds differently to altitude, and what feels fine for one person can feel unpleasantly exhausting for another.

Stay hydrated. At altitude we lose water via our lungs even when we're not sweating, so keep drinking (water). Steer clear of alcohol while acclimatizing—or restrict yourself to a small glass of wine in the evenings.

Wear layers—it's often colder as you climb higher. Choose fabrics that wick away moisture, and ditch the cotton T-shirts (or anything made of cotton).

Weather at altitude is often unpredictable. Keep an eye on the forecast, and take waterproof clothing if need be.

UV rays are more intense, risking damage to the eyes, so wear sunglasses and use appropriate sunscreen.

Don't carry more than you need. Walking at altitude can feel more tiring than walking at sea level, so pack accordingly and pace yourself.

For long, demanding ascents, use the Afghan walking technique in Week 35: Walk Like a Nomad (p. 144).

Always take a map, and never rely on your phone, which may not work in remote areas!

Not everyone experiences altitude sickness, but a few people suffer at heights as low as 2,000 meters, so know the signs: headache, nausea, dizziness, severe shortness of breath. And be prepared to descend immediately.

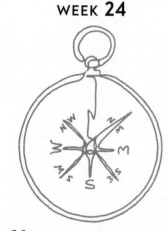

Walk with a Map

IN SEPTEMBER 1924 AN EIGHTEEN-YEAR-OLD girl tucked herself under some old pages of *Le Monde* newspaper and curled up beneath the Pont Saint-Michel in Paris's Latin Quarter. Although drunks and outcasts settled down beside her, Phyllis Pearsall ignored them, focusing instead on the map she was building in her head. She had come to stay with her brother. But her brother had disappeared—and without money, friends, or family, Phyllis had nowhere to go.

Phyllis had no map of Paris, either, but she had seen and memorized one, sketching it in her head and then drawing and redrawing it in her mind's eye. She used this memory map to find her way around Paris, learning to tell the time and recognize her whereabouts by sniffing at the Paris air: bread and chocolat chaud in the morning; chicken and galettes at midday; frying fish, garlic, lamb, and tarte Tatin in the evening. Later Phyllis became one of the world's most successful mapmakers, creating the first A–Z map of London and founding the Geographers' A–Z Map Company.

Phyllis worked until she died, a month short of her ninetieth birthday. She's a testament to what neuroscientists have since learned: that every walk is an opportunity to grow our brain. And the simplest and easiest way to do this is to walk with a paper map. Straying from your usual route, guided only by a paper or a mental map, will quite literally expand your mind.

Neuroscience suggests that the hippocampus, the part of our brain used for navigation, grows as we use it and withers when we don't—a sort of use-it-or-lose-it navigational muscle. Studies of London cabdrivers famously found them in possession of impressively large posterior hippocampi, thanks to the navigational demands of learning the whereabouts of every London street. Alas, satellite navigation systems have put an end to this. According to the navigation expert David Barrie, our reliance on technology is not only shrinking essential parts of our brains, but also leaving us prone to Alzheimer's and dementia. People with Alzheimer's have notoriously poor (often absent) navigational skills: I have vivid memories of my grandmother wandering around, unable to recognize where she was.

Why does this happen, and how can walking prevent it? Our hippocampus acts as the storage container for all the place memories we've ever had. Whenever we visit somewhere new, we create a spatial memory, which is then stored in a series of cells known as place, grid, and border cells. The details are located on a place map and stored in our hippocampus. When we visit a new location, our place maps reorganize themselves, creating a brand-new map in the process. Think of it as a giant filing system that we can borrow from whenever we need to. In that filing system is every home we've lived in; every office we've worked in; the route we took to school; and the surrounding roads, fields and parks, all neatly filed and ready for retrieval. Moreover, these maps are uniquely ours, encoded using our own criteria.

It's a mind-bogglingly impressive construction, well worth preserving, not only because without it we are physically and spatially lost, but because our place memories are intrinsic to our identity. Our sense of self is often rooted in the places we've inhabited. When we lose our place memories, we lose an essential part of ourselves.

To boot, researchers now speculate that the regions of our brain responsible for spatial navigation also play a part in other more conceptual types of navigation, like prediction, imagination, and creativity, where we use our mind's eye to help make decisions. Some researchers suspect that the same brain regions may also be involved in social navigation, helping us navigate interpersonal relationships. The message is clear: when our place cells atrophy, so does the rest of us.

Being shepherded everywhere by technology has many benefits, but brain-building isn't one of them. So take a map (and a waterproof map holder if it's raining), turn the phone off, and start walking.

When I take map walks, I start with a rough idea of my destination but no set timings. (This is neither a getting-lost walk—see Week 41, p. 170—nor a race.) Cities are particularly good because they offer multiple routes, and the mere process of selecting a route places additional demands on the brain. Invest plenty of time in map gazing before you depart—you need a rough idea of direction, an approximate idea of how long it might take to walk, and ideally a route free of arterial roads. When you start walking, pay particular attention to landmarks, the critical locators that will help you return, or find the route again, with or without a map. Studies suggest we find larger landmarks more helpful, so think church steeples and tall trees rather than trash bins and bushes. Landmarks that are personally meaningful are also more likely to persist in our memory: my children never fail to recall the locations of bakeries and ice-cream shops, for example.

Using visual landmarks to spatially locate ourselves is known as landmark-based piloting. But to work our brains still harder, we need to include all our senses. Researchers now believe that human beings have a highly developed sense of smell, much greater than once thought. In recent experiments, blindfolded students followed scent trails while on their hands and knees—with staggering success. As you walk (upright, not on all fours), sniff out factories, gas stations, bakeries, trees. Use your ears in the same way, committing to memory any locational sounds. Refer to your map in order to locate yourself and—if you want—to cross-reference landmarks, smells, and sounds with your geographical position.

In the countryside you may want to borrow from the excellent navigational work of Tristan Gooley, who uses natural signs to locate and navigate himself. Who knew that we can take our bearings from the heights of trees? Or that lichen can be used to orient ourselves?

Map walks are excellent when accompanied by children, not only because they appreciate the inherent adventure but because—thanks to on-screen childhoods and growing parental concerns with safety—children are at the greatest risk of losing their navigational brain muscle. Whoever you're with, share the map reading and navigation so that all can benefit.

TIPS

IT'S MORE DIFFICULT TO SELF-ORIENT in the countryside: take a compass or use the compass on your phone.

While city map walks can begin with a destination in mind, these are less obvious in the country. Country map walks that choose and follow a footpath, rather than heading for an end point, are just as effective at building our navigational brain muscle.

Walking with children? Delegate—without question—stretches of map reading and be prepared to follow where they lead.

Whether you're in an urban or rural area, try returning without using your map.

Above all, resist the temptation to defer to Google Maps (or the moving dot on apps like AllTrails) until absolutely necessary.

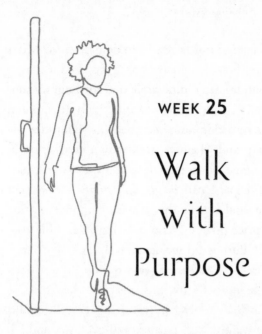

WEEK **25**

Walk with Purpose

THE CELEBRATED FRENCH COMPOSER ERIK Satie walked daily from his home to his studio—a six-mile walk across Paris that he repeated, in reverse, at the end of each day. His walk passed through a straggle of notoriously dangerous streets. To protect himself, Satie carried a hammer. He walked with speed and determination, composing in his head even as he watched out for his safety. I like to think that Satie's brisk, purposeful walking helped counter his absinthe habit, enabling him to compose famously innovative music until he died.

Today, researchers refer to Satie's style of bipedalism or movement as *utilitarian walking* or simply *walking with purpose*. The human need for a sense of purpose has been found, repeatedly, to define how we see ourselves: purpose gives our lives meaning. Numerous studies attest to the power of purpose for keeping us engaged, curious, and fulfilled. As we live, so can we walk. A sense of *walking purpose* helps us pick up our pace, encouraging us to walk, like Satie, both farther and faster. In so doing, we *feel* better and healthier.

Everyone loves a Sunday-afternoon stroll, and many of us happily drive to a local trail or park in order to amble with friends and family. Walks like this provide numerous benefits, but when we walk from our doorstep and when we walk with a destination in mind, be it the office, home, or an appointment, we also participate in what public health experts call *incidental activity*—movement that forms part of our regular day rather than something requiring a specific time slot or place (like "exercise" needing an evening class at a gym, for example). Purposeful incidental walking—like Satie's daily on-foot commute—is the easiest way to increase our daily steps. It may also be the most effective in terms of our health.

A study from Ohio State University involving 125,000 adults found that those who walked with purpose walked faster and felt healthier than those who walked solely for recreation. Walking of all types made people feel better, regardless of the duration or purpose, explained associate professor Gulsah Akar. "But walking for utilitarian purposes significantly improves health."

Akar found that people walking with purpose—to work, to shop, or to an appointment—walked faster than those who walked for leisure. It may be this additional speed that makes us feel healthier. Akar found that walking to work in particular resulted in faster walking and greater reported health.

When we ditch the car and do more of our everyday journeys on foot, not only do we walk with greater vigor but we also clock up extra minutes of exercise. Akar's study found that when we walk directly from our house ("walking trips that begin at home"), we walk for longer and at greater speed, giving us "significantly greater . . . health." It's an argument that walking coach Joanna Hall makes: "Having a few walks that start from the front door are absolutely essential, even very short ones—we always walk at an accelerated pace when we know the route, and if it's on our doorstep it's much harder to procrastinate." For many of us this may be because our immediate locality feels dully familiar or involves hazardous road walking, prompting us to speed up. Or it may be because quotidian walking often has to be squeezed into busy days.

Either way, it's not difficult to add purposeful walking into our lives. Try leaving the car behind whenever you have an appointment or social occasion within walking distance. Don't be too generous with time: you want to be striding, not dawdling.

Evening strolls and afternoon ambles can also be done with purpose. Start from your house rather than driving—the familiar home stretch will invariably be walked more quickly—and set a time limit or a reason to be home at a certain time. A stew that needs to be removed from the oven, a TV program, or just an alarm on your phone—almost anything can double as a purpose-inducing deadline.

TIPS

TO PICK UP SPEED, LEAVE fractionally later but keep the same time goal.

Find alternatives to dangerously fast and polluted roads, seeking out backstreets and footpaths wherever possible. Navigation apps like Go Jauntly are much better at identifying walking routes than more traffic-oriented apps.

Don't let the familiarity of your usual habitat urge you into your car—even walks we perceive as dull can become interesting if we use some of the other tips in this book (by using our nose, for example—see Week 11: Take a City Smell Walk, p. 44).

Listening to audiobooks and podcasts can transform utilitarian walking into something genuinely interesting. Keep one earpiece out if you're near traffic.

Start from your front door: the monotony of a known landscape encourages acceleration.

Unable to walk safely from your doorstep? Lobby your elected representative for walkable paths, more green space, or legislation that curbs pollution and reduces the speed of traffic.

Other ways of building purposeful walking into our lives include training for a walking marathon or step tracking. Studies show that reluctant walkers who track their step count typically walk farther and for longer.

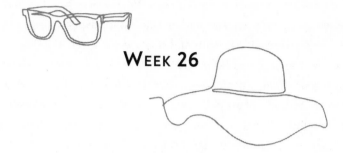

WEEK 26

Walk in Sunshine

SUN WORSHIP HAS EXISTED FOR millennia, but it wasn't until a little-known Danish scientist began observing a local cat that light became recognized as a force for good health. Niels Ryberg Finsen's interest in heliotherapy was rooted in his own debilitating sickness, a metabolic disease that was to kill him at the age of forty-four. Twenty years earlier, as a medical student, he noticed how sunshine rejuvenated him. Watching cats gravitate to sunny spots encouraged him to experiment more intensively on himself, strengthening his conviction that "the sun had a useful and important effect."

Finsen later won the 1903 Nobel Prize for his light-therapy work, in particular for his success with smallpox and lupus vulgaris, a form of tuberculosis. Word of his achievements spread, and thirty-six heliotherapy centers (sometimes called sunbathing clinics or solaria) were built in the Swiss Alps by the best-known heliotherapist, Dr. Auguste Rollier. Under Rollier's care, patients were slowly—and often with superb results—exposed to sunlight, starting with as little as five minutes of early morning sun on their feet. Unsurprisingly, tans became fashionable, a sign not only of wealth but of health, inspiring the editor of *The Times* to boldly assert that "days of darkness are also days of death and disease."

Today we avoid the sun, and many of us spend the best part of our days in artificial light. Thanks to our increasingly indoor lifestyle, our zealous use of sunscreen, our obsessive fear of wrinkles, and rising levels of air pollution, up to 70 percent of the population is thought be deficient in sunlight's best known by-product, vitamin D. Scientists unraveling the near-miraculous qualities of sunshine now think that vitamin D is only one of its remarkable benefits. As Finsen suspected, we need the full rays of the sun. For those of us living in northern latitudes, stepping out at every dazzling glimmer of light makes perfect sense.

Vitamin D remains hugely important. Created when the ultraviolet light (UVB) in sunshine hits our skin, it travels to our liver and on to our kidneys before finally morphing into a hormone called calcidiol, 25(OH)D. Calcidiol lasts between two and three weeks, so our bodies need continuous sunshine in order to keep our serum levels stable. Experts recommend between five and thirty minutes of light on the face, neck, and arms every day, depending on skin type and UV index.

The pivotal role of vitamin D leaped to prominence during the COVID-19 pandemic, when low levels of it were linked to poorer recovery, and when it became apparent that—somehow—it was crucial to the functioning of our innate immune system. It's now thought that we have two immune systems: innate and acquired. Our acquired immunity develops as we're exposed to pathogens, a process that triggers the production of antibodies (and the process by which vaccines work). Our innate immunity is the defense system already built into our bodies, enabling us to deal with everyday exposure to germs, allergens, and so on. Our innate immune system is responsible for fending off many viruses. Links between our innate immunity and vitamin D indicated that adequate serum levels could hold the key to keeping wintertime viruses like the flu and common cold at bay, a finding supported by numerous other studies.

But here's the thing: vitamin D isn't the only benefit of sunlight, which explains why supplementation hasn't always been effective. Heart disease, hypertension, osteoporosis, several cancers, depression, dementia, and multiple autoimmune diseases have recently been linked to a deficiency not of vitamin D, but of sunshine. A two-decade Swedish study of 30,000 women identified a dramatically higher rate of death among sun-avoiders. Its author claimed that lack of sunlight was as dangerous for our health as smoking, pleading for "a more balanced and adequate view regarding the effects of sun exposure on our health."

So could sunlight be the long-sought elixir of life? Researchers now believe photons from sunlight activate our T cells, vital components of our immune system sometimes called defender cells, by mobilizing nitric oxide from our skin and transferring it into our circulatory system. Our skin carries a large number of T cells— twice as many as those circulating in our blood. The blue light in sunshine reaches not only the surface layer of our skin but also the layer below (the dermis), enabling rapid activation of the vast swaths of T cells lurking there. "Sunlight directly activates key immune cells by increasing their movement," explained researcher Gerard Ahern at Georgetown University Medical Center.

To boot, sunlight plays a critical role in setting our circadian rhythms and moderating our production of melatonin, thereby helping us to wake and sleep. None of these are anything to do with vitamin D, meaning that avoiding sunshine and relying on a supplement instead may be monumentally stupid.

The tangled subjects of sunlight and vitamin D remain contentious. Researchers still argue about how much vitamin D and/or sunlight we need. Some believe high-dose supplements interfere with the delicate workings of our microbiome, while many oncologists and dermatologists maintain that we should forgo all sun and rely on supplementation alone.

It sounds complicated, but the answer is simple: take a short walk whenever the sun shines, sleeves rolled up, skin free of sunscreen. In my own self-experimentation, six months of careful sun-exposed walking nudged me into remission from an autoimmune disease and led to a winter entirely free of coughs and colds.

The last word should go to the British surgeon and heliotherapist Henry Gauvain, who described sunlight as "like a good champagne. It invigorates and stimulates; indulged in to excess, it intoxicates and poisons."

TIPS

WALK ON THE SUNNY SIDE of the path or street, beside water if you can. (The reflections provide additional UV light.)

Short of time? Go at midday, when the UVB rays are at their most intense.

Always avoid burning by covering up after between ten and thirty minutes, according to your skin type, your location, and the time of day and year. Set a timer on your phone or watch. When it goes off, cover up with clothes, shade, and/or sunscreen.

Prepare your body for weaker winter immunity and low levels of winter sunlight by snatching every autumn opportunity for a sunny walk.

Avoid walking in heavily polluted areas: studies of Indian children, Middle Eastern young women, and Belgian postmenopausal women found that high levels of atmospheric pollution "significantly" reduced the amount of UVB, raising the risk of vitamin D deficiency.

Know the benefits of morning sunlight for setting your circadian rhythms and improving your nighttime sleep (see Week 10: Walk Within an Hour of Waking, p. 40).

Concerned about exposing your skin to the sun without sunscreen? Prepare your skin slowly, building exposure incrementally. Check with your physician if you're concerned, but never let your skin burn.

Alternatively, invest in one of the new mineral sunscreens that protect us from harmful UV rays without depriving us of vitamin D and nitric oxide.

Too bright to look up? A wide-brimmed hat or cap helps maintain posture.

Ever wondered why you feel better when the sun shines? In addition to everything else, sunlight also triggers the feel-good hormone serotonin. The brighter the light, the greater the levels of serotonin, according to a study in *The Lancet*.

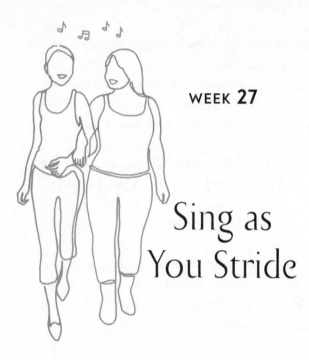

Sing as You Stride

ONE DAMP AUTUMNAL MORNING IN 1854, the writer and walker George Borrow set off to climb Snowdon, the highest mountain in Wales. In his customary black suit, an umbrella under his elbow, he linked arms with his companion—his stepdaughter, Henrietta— and sang Welsh songs at the top of his voice until they reached the summit. Why? Because he was worried that Henrietta, being a woman, might not manage such an arduous hike. He was also worried that Henrietta (being a woman) might feel frightened. Either way, she needed strengthening with song.

Mr. Borrow understood intuitively what scientists have since proved using mood scales, stress scales, blood tests, saliva tests, and brain scans: the bonding, fortifying, and energizing power of song. Singing while walking has been used tactically throughout history— by marching soldiers, hiking schoolchildren, dissenting protesters, and . . . weary families. We made full use of it on our first family hiking holiday in the Austrian Alps. As the slopes became steeper, our songs became louder. And, like Mr. Borrow and Henrietta, we reached the summits in record time.

What is it about singing that helps us climb mountains? The physiological benefits are well documented. Singing dulls pain, something medics attribute to a series of neurochemicals released when we break into song, including beta-endorphins that act as natural painkillers.

Singing provides our lungs with a workout, resulting in enhanced respiratory muscles and more efficient breathing. Researchers call this *optimized breathing*, and arguably, it's exactly what we need as we walk, particularly if we sing in rhythm with our feet. When we open our lungs to sing, we involuntarily improve our posture, and when we exhale, we reduce muscle tension. Singing is aerobic: like walking, it pumps oxygen into the blood, making us feel invigorated and uplifted.

When we sing, we also strengthen our immune system. Study after study has found raised levels of an immune-boosting antibody called immunoglobulin A (IgA) in the saliva of singers—that's you, me, and anyone else who enjoys a good singsong.

When the writer Katharine Trevelyan crossed Canada in 1935, alone and on foot, she sang to calm herself. Saliva tests have since proven that singing relaxes us by reducing our levels of cortisol, the fight-or-flight hormone that in excess contributes to stress, depression, insomnia, and heart disease.

Evidence for the psychological effects of singing is equally convincing. In cancer patients and their caregivers, in psychiatric patients, in elderly people with dementia, in pregnant mothers, in nursing staff, and in students, dozens of studies have established that singing produces endorphins, making us feel happier. Much of the research has focused on choirs, but one study compared the benefits of singing alone with those of group singing and found no difference. Anyone who sings produces feel-good endorphins, regardless of who they're with and where they are. As one researcher wrote, with stark brevity, happiness was increased and worry and sadness were reduced after both choir and solo singing.

And yet singing with others brings additional perks. It pulls us outside of ourselves, encouraging us to coordinate rhythm, melody, and lyrics with our companions. Instantly we think of other people rather than ourselves, but—crucially—we also perceive ourselves as part of a group. Scientists think this triggers another neurochemical: oxytocin, known as the friendship, empathy, or bonding chemical. As our brain floods with oxytocin, we feel what neuroscientist Daniel Levitin, author of *This Is Your Brain on Music*, describes as a real bond and sense of trust and well-being toward those we're singing with.

Reports of stroke survivors and Parkinson's patients show that singing while walking also helps with rehabilitation. Both groups of patients often find their walking style significantly disrupted: shortened steps, difficulty balancing, an uneven stride, and painfully slow movements mean many can walk only a short distance with the help of a cane. A Korean experiment involving stroke survivors between the ages of nineteen and seventy-eight yielded dramatic results. As the stroke survivors walked, they sang a nursery rhyme, chosen because its tempo range of 90 to 120 beats per minute made it an ideal walking speed. Within thirty minutes the participants were moving more evenly, with longer strides and greater speed. A study of Parkinson's patients had similar results—singing while walking led to greater improvements than any other intervention. This happens because the parts of our brain that control our movements also control our ability to maintain a steady rhythm.

So what holds us back from singing as we walk? Levitin points the finger at an inhibition circuit in our brain that continually nudges us into behaving "appropriately," by making us feel repressingly self-conscious when we act foolishly. It's also the brain part affected by alcohol, which explains why a few drinks can make us feel joyously and recklessly uninhibited.

So we could swig from a hip flask on our walks, hoping the alcohol will release us from "social propriety." Or we could coax our walking companions into singing along—children will be delighted. Alternatively, we could stop fretting and simply break into song, knowing that our immunity will be improved, our spirits lifted, our gait emboldened, our companion ties strengthened . . . and the mountain summit reached. Nor is lack of talent any reason to hold back. Musicologists believe most of us can hold a tune, particularly when singing in a group.

TIPS

CHOOSE A SONG THAT EVERYONE knows or can learn in a few minutes. Check that it has the right tempo, although any toe-tapping melody will work.

If the lyrics fit, all the better: we like the folk song "She'll Be Coming Round the Mountain."

Don't expect to see wildlife if you're singing your hearts out.

The reverse works too. A loud tune will keep away snakes, bears, and other unwelcome visitors.

Be sensitive to other walkers who may not wish to hear your dulcet tones ringing through the valley.

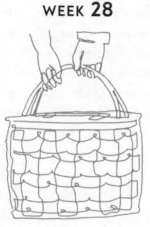

Walk with a Picnic

SOMETIME AROUND 1858—BETWEEN THE DEATH of her first baby and the birth of her second—the cookbook writer Mrs. Isabella Beeton wrote out a picnic menu. It included:

> a joint of cold roast beef, a joint of cold boiled beef,
> 2 ribs of lamb, 2 shoulders of lamb, 4 roast fowls, 2 roast
> duck, 1 ham, 1 tongue, 2 veal and ham pies, 2 pigeon
> pies, 6 medium lobsters, 1 piece of collared calves
> head, 18 lettuces, 6 baskets of salad, 6 cucumbers . . .
> 2 dozen fruit turnovers, 4 dozen cheese cakes, 2 cold
> cabinet puddings in molds, 1 large cold Christmas
> pudding, a few baskets of fresh fruit . . .

And this was before she got to the breads, cakes, cheeses, butter (6 pounds), and drinks!

Carrying all this to a remote picnic spot (and then lugging back the bones, leftovers, cutlery, and crockery, not to mention the napkins and cloths that Mrs. Beeton deemed essential) would test the muscles and stamina of any hiker.

But *carrying* was something our ancestors did, hour after hour and day after day. When we carry objects, our muscles engage in isometric contractions—extended contractions quite different from those involved in a bicep curl, for instance. When we walk with a picnic hamper, the muscles in our arms, shoulders, and core contract and stay contracted until we put the hamper down. This builds strength in our muscles without impacting our joints—because our joints don't move.

There are three types of muscle contraction: concentric—the shortening of a muscle that takes place when we lift a weight; eccentric—the lengthening of a muscle that takes place as we lower a weight; and isometric—the holding of a muscle for a prolonged period. Although all three work as a team, supporting and stabilizing our limbs, isometric movement is particularly adept at maintaining muscle strength, endurance, and mobility. Today few of us regularly engage in the sort of activities that involve isometric muscle contraction. But recent studies suggest that isometric exercise works 95 percent of a muscle, as opposed to the 88 to 90 percent worked during eccentric and concentric contractions. Some sports scientists believe isometric exercise builds greater strength than lifting and lowering weights (where the emphasis is on concentric and eccentric contractions).

Isometric exercises are often used in rehabilitation programs, where joints must be kept stress-free but muscle needs to be rebuilt or maintained. Exercise involving isometric contracting is also very useful for people who enjoy yoga, cross-country skiing, climbing, and ballet—where strong muscles are needed to hold a position.

The combination of walking and carrying (sometimes referred to as *loading* or *loaded carry*) is infinitely more complex than lifting a dumbbell. Our bodies need to remain stable and balanced with every step, while our brains have to calculate how best to move with something that might not be uniformly shaped. The muscles in our arms, shoulders, abdominals, and core are thoroughly put to work when we carry a Mrs. Beeton–style picnic.

Which is what happened to the diarist Ellen Weeton and the four men who helped carry her picnic on July 8, 1810, as they walked "for five or six miles . . . along a very rocky rugged path . . . over moss and rocks" to reach the summit of Fairfield Fell in England's Lake District, carrying "veal, ham, chicken, gooseberry pies, bread, cheese, butter, hung leg of mutton, wine, porter, rum, brandy and bitters." Their walk—"eight or ten miles . . . some say twelve"—carrying a heavy spread, much of it "scrambled" over "rocks, mountain heath and moss," required prolonged muscle contractions, building strength and endurance and improving balance.

In the past it was perfectly normal to carry as you walked. There was no need for hand or ankle weights when people routinely carried baskets of produce, buckets of water, small children, suitcases, rucksacks made of canvas and leather with heavy brass buckles. In 1914, the writer Mary Webb and her husband walked ten miles every Saturday carrying enormous armfuls of garden produce that they sold at the local market. At the age of seventy-three, the walker and businessman William Hutton walked twenty-eight miles a day with a billycan of water, an umbrella, maps, notebooks, pens, and ink bottles—a load he considered light but which in all likelihood weighed many pounds.

Which is not to say we all need to be carting lavish picnics up and down mountains. My point is this: our muscles are designed not only to lift objects and put them down but *to carry them for sustained periods*. When we don't use our muscles in this way, they atrophy, ultimately resulting in sarcopenia—muscles so withered and wasted we cannot get up from a chair. Indeed, some strength coaches think load-carrying is the single most effective way to build strength. They're thinking of sandbags rather than picnic baskets, but let's not split hairs.

Picnicking was a favorite pastime when my children were young. They found walking dull, but transformed into an expedition with a picnic at the end, a walk became an adventure—because all food tastes immeasurably better outside, whatever the weather. We have picnicked under bushes in the rain, deep in forests among myriad insects, in city parks and cemeteries, in summer and in winter. None of our picnics were to Mrs. Beeton's standard, but neither did they weigh as much.

Instead of pumping iron at the gym, put together a picnic, invite a few friends, and walk. As you labor beneath your load, think not only of the gastronomic pleasures to come but of your muscles, stronger and more powerful than ever. There's something incredibly liberating about knowing you could carry someone down a hill if you needed to.

TIPS

TAKE ONLY WHAT YOU CAN comfortably carry.

Hold your load/picnic basket close to your waist and use both arms, so the weight is evenly distributed. (This is sometimes called a sandbag carry or a bear-hug carry.) Alternatively, use what's known as a farmer's walk (something in each hand) or a suitcase carry (carried like an old-fashioned case, swapping arms regularly).

Bend from the legs when you pick up (and put down), not from your waist.

Change direction from your feet, not from your torso.

Keep your spine straight, and engage your core to protect your back.

Don't fret about carrying in one hand. Research shows that if one arm only is used, the brain sends a message to the noncarrying arm instructing its muscle to stay strong . . . a sort of workout by proxy, and another example of how mind-bogglingly miraculous our bodies are.

Walking a long way? Put some of the picnic on your back (see Week 36: Walk with a Pack, p. 148). This makes it easier to carry and leaves your hands free.

If you're including a picnic with a night/rainy/windy walk, prepare accordingly (hot and easy for the night, quick and simple for rain, warm and weighty for wind).

The best picnics include something a little surprising. Forget the sandwiches and chips: search online or browse specialized picnic books.

Alternatively—although not half as much fun—use a resistance band as you walk. Harvard fitness consultant Michele Stanten suggests working your chest, arm, or shoulder muscles by stretching the band while holding it in front of or above you. Otherwise, loop it around your upper body and push it forward with your arms as you walk.

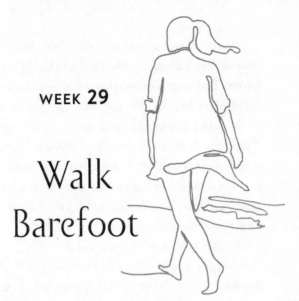

WEEK **29**

Walk
Barefoot

A HUNDRED YEARS AGO, BAREFOOT walking was a popular pursuit among a small, health-conscious contingent of the British population. James Bain, a Scottish minister and founder of the Barefoot League, argued that, "All parts of the earth's surface on which we tread will fulfill a particular service of life for the health of the body." Bain believed that our feet absorbed the goodness of the land, taking its nutrients directly into our bloodstream. Although his barefoot walking began in the Scottish countryside, he continued the habit "on the pavements of London and . . . Edinburgh," unable to forgo the exhilarating freedom he felt shoeless, the way his body became "simply aglow with radiant energy."

At a summer school in Brighton, Bain introduced barefoot walking to young men and women, leading a daily two-mile barefoot walk from the school to the beach. He was delighted with the results: "Very soon their bodies were charged through and through with the most potent of all physical vivifiers . . . really wondrous effects in the beauty of health were soon evident to all who had seeing eyes."

There's growing evidence that John Bain may have been onto something all along. In his studies of footfall, evolutionary biologist Daniel Lieberman found that wearing cushioned shoes causes us to tread more heavily, putting huge additional pressure on our knee joints. "The energy that gets shot up your leg is about three times bigger in a cushioned shoe than if you're barefoot," he says. Lieberman believes this extra impact may explain why rates of knee arthritis have doubled in the last seventy years, precisely the time period in which technological advances gifted us cushioned soles. Cushioned footwear, he adds, may be affecting our balance, leaving us vulnerable to falls as we grow older.

Lieberman is not alone in his concerns. A 2007 study compared modern feet to those of 2,000-year-old skeletons and found our barefoot ancestors had healthier and better-formed feet. Later, researchers found that forgoing footwear improved knee osteoarthritis, reversed back pain, and positively altered gait.

The spotlight recently extended to toe springs, the upward curve on the toes of most athletic shoes. The first report to investigate them made the point that although toe springs add to the ease and comfort of walking, they too are weakening our feet, rendering us susceptible to painful foot conditions like plantar fasciitis. The authors noted that "weak intrinsic foot muscles are an evolutionary mismatch caused by the foot not being entirely adapted for modern shoes" whose "arch supports, cushioning, and other supportive features . . . increase comfort and reduce the work that the foot muscles have to do."

It appears that our feet—and the twenty-six bones, thirty-three joints, and nineteen muscles they contain—may not appreciate the luxury and ease of modern footwear as much as we do.

When we walk barefoot, we walk differently, landing more lightly, with less of a heel thump and with our weight more evenly distributed. Studies suggest that without shoes we walk more slowly and with a shorter stride, but that we also take a greater number of steps. More interesting, we open ourselves to an extraordinary range of sensations previously lost on our thick-soled boots or ultra-cushioned sneakers. Our feet have almost twice as many nerve endings as a penis, making them one of the most intensely tactile and sensuous parts of our body. For me, this is the great delight of barefoot walking—soft sand, dewy grass, cropped turf, moist moss, sun-warmed stone, and countless other sensations make it clear why John Bain returned from his walks aglow with radiant energy.

Being barefoot changes our experience of walking. Not only do we move differently, but we feel oddly rooted, aware of a new universe beneath our feet. This is 360-degree walking—and it's joyful.

TIPS

SANDY BEACHES, GRASSY MOUNTAIN SLOPES, and mossy forest floors are the perfect spots to investigate barefoot walking.

In cities, cemeteries make ideal locations. Parks with dog-free zones are similarly clean. Otherwise, walk barefoot around your home and garden.

Seek out local barefoot parks or trails. Germany is the spiritual home of barefoot walking, with dozens of routes, while Brazil's Lençóis Maranhenses National Park is ideal for multiday barefoot treks.

Minimal or minimalist footwear—with its thinner sole, paucity of cushioning, and wider toe box—offers a perfect compromise: the protection of a shoe without the potentially damaging cushioning, arch support, and toe springs of modern sneakers. Research suggests this type of footwear can strengthen the arches and muscles of our feet in the same way as barefoot walking.

Note that habitual barefoot walking will widen your feet—be prepared for a wardrobe of shoes that no longer fit!

Worried that hardened, calloused soles will destroy the sensitivity in your feet? They won't: studies show that hardened barefoot walkers experience identical sensations, despite their thickened skin.

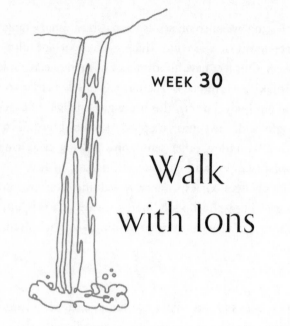

WEEK **30**

Walk with Ions

DURING THE SPRING OF 1802, the poet Samuel Taylor Coleridge plunged into the darkest depression of his life. Coleridge was familiar with despair, its bleak corners and its hopeless cul-de-sacs. But he also knew that—in the right landscape—he could outwalk his "Darkness & Dimness . . . [the] bewildering Shame, and Pain that is utterly Lord over us."

Coleridge, already a seasoned walker, began taking ever-lengthier hikes. For eighteen months he walked at every opportunity: alone, up and down craggy mountains, through mud-bound woods, beside dashing streams. He walked in pearly sunshine, but he also walked—with considerable enthusiasm—in driving rain and through stinging sleet.

Most significantly, however, he walked to and from waterfalls. The writer Robert Macfarlane, in his account of Coleridge's sudden fascination for waterfalls, explains that "if there was any purpose in [Coleridge's] mind, it seems to have been to join up the waterfalls of the land around him." Coleridge called them "great water-slopes" and dreamed of creating his own waterfall map. His waterfall walks, often taken in a "hard storm of rain," were the most consoling and inspiring of all his walks during this dark, turbulent time in his life.

Scientists now have a possible explanation for the healing power of Coleridge's rain-blown waterfall walks: negative air ions. Breaking water surfaces disrupt air molecules, splitting them, mixing them with water molecules, and charging (ionizing) them with electricity in the process—thereby turning them into air ions. Air ions are either positively (generally less good for us) or negatively (generally good for us) charged, according to whether electrons or protons predominate. Positive ions are heavier and typically fall to the ground. Negative ions—which carry an extra negative charge—are small and light, enabling them to stay airborne.

This process is exaggerated around waterfalls, where the colossal force of tumbling water fractures water droplets in a very special way, creating an abundance of nanoparticles that hover, mistily and exuberantly, in the air. Scientists first discovered the special air around waterfalls over a hundred years ago and now call it the *waterfall effect*.

When a team of Austrian researchers embarked on a two-year study of waterfall air, carefully and repeatedly measuring the ions at five separate waterfalls, they discovered that the negative ion count often reached several tens of thousands per cubic centimeter, an astonishingly rich density that was up to 120 times higher than normal outdoor air.

But can exposure to waterfalls really improve our mood and health? Earlier studies revealed that asthmatic children who spent an hour a day playing near a waterfall lessened their symptoms, strengthened their lungs, improved their immunity, and reduced their levels of inflammation. But could these results be replicated among healthy adults?

To investigate more fully, another team of Austrian scientists recruited ninety stressed care workers and put them into three groups. The first group spent an hour a day beside a waterfall as part of their hiking route. The second group hiked away from waterfalls. A third (control) group continued with their regular lives. After a week, both hiking groups had lowered heart rates and greatly reduced stress. But a battery of tests revealed that the waterfall group had—on almost every count—significantly less psychological distress, impressively improved lung capacity, and considerably higher levels of a vital antibody called secretory immunoglobulin A (SIgA). SIgA—found in the mucosal lining of our nostrils, gut, and mouth—is a crucial first line of defense in our immune system, protecting us from dozens of pathogens and toxins ranging from coronaviruses to air pollution. To the scientists' surprise, the waterfall group continued to show improved immunity, with raised levels of SIgA, eight weeks later.

Their findings reflected those from earlier experiments on mice and rats, in which water-generated negative ions improved the rodents' immunity, prompting the Austrian researchers to ponder whether the waterfalls' abundant negative ions might be penetrating our skin and mucosal surfaces (inside our noses and mouths, for example), altering our microbiota, and creating a "waterfall-altered microbiome," which in turn might account for the participants' stronger immunity.

Could a waterfall's microbiological atmosphere—in which nature's microbes and phytoncides are blended and diffused through mists of negative ions—be a miracle pill for the mind and body? Scientists don't yet have an answer. But Coleridge found one: his depression duly lifted, replaced by "a fantastic Pleasure, that draws the soul along." Eva Selhub and Alan Logan provide corroborating evidence in their book *Your Brain on Nature*: exposure to negative ions improves health, cognition, and longevity, while making us more relaxed and less depressed, stressed, and anxious.

Meanwhile, research picked up pace during COVID-19, when investigations revealed that negative air ions were capable of deactivating coronaviruses. Experiments carried out at the University of Oklahoma—using negative ion generators rather than waterfalls—enabled scientists to observe the way in which negative air ions attached to the positively charged protein at the end of a coronaviral spike, effectively neutralizing it. Negative ion generators have also had success in laboratory trials on people with seasonal depression, where thirty-minute daily sessions dramatically improved mood.

Negative ions exist in a delicate and complex web of conditions and factors, and research continues to shed light on them. But one thing is certain: indoor air has the lowest negative ion count. So forget the gym and go outside. But it's not merely "count" that matters: negative air ions have varying life spans. Urban ions survive for only a few seconds, while forest, ocean, and waterfall ions can live for up to twenty minutes.

TIPS

THE AUSTRIAN RESEARCHERS NOTED THAT ion concentrations fluctuated, depending on the weight or force of flowing water—during spring snowmelt or a drenching downpour, ion counts were at their highest. Seek out ferociously colliding water in wet, stormy weather—as Coleridge did—and spend at least thirty minutes lapping up its wild music and its invigorating ions.

Studies suggest that mountains have the highest overall levels of negative air ions: seek out waterfalls in mountainous regions, if you can.

Misty spring morning? Head to a forest. Forests and woodlands are also spectacularly high in negative air ions—double that of open land, particularly when leaves are forming, or during mist, when negative air ions linger in the air.

A wild-water swim with plenty of splashing creates a microbiological atmosphere akin (almost) to a waterfall. Find a walking route with a wild swimming spot.

Waves exploding on a shoreline imbue coastal air with negative ions: walk as closely as you (safely) dare to seething surf.

Racing rivers—like those in spate—also trigger large volumes of ions (see Week 17: Follow a River, p. 67).

Cities generally suffer from a dearth of negative ions, so look for any moving water—fountains, water features, or rivers.

Negative ions increase when rain falls. The heavier the rain, the greater the number of negative ions, although this levels off after a while. Walk in a downpour—wherever you are (see Week 12: Walk in the Rain, p. 48).

Negative air ions are typically at their highest concentration from midnight through early morning, peaking between seven and eleven A.M., decreasing at noon, and gradually increasing in the evening. An early morning walk (see Week 10: Walk Within an Hour of Waking, p. 40), night walk (see Week 46: Take a Night Walk, p. 190), or an evening stroll (see Week 42: Walk After Eating, p. 173) will maximize negative air ion exposure.

Negative air ions occur all year round, but studies show they have a preference for summer and autumn. They also linger for longer in clean air.

Meteorological factors greatly affect the prevalence and abundance of negative ions. They lessen on long, sunny days; increase on windy and stormy days; loiter in humid conditions; slink away in urban fog. Try a windy walk (see Week 9: Take a Windy Walk, p. 36).

UV rays also create negative ions (see Week 26: Walk in Sunshine, p. 105), as do thunderstorms, when the combined "charge" of vast quantities of ionized molecules can make the air quite literally sizzle with electricity.

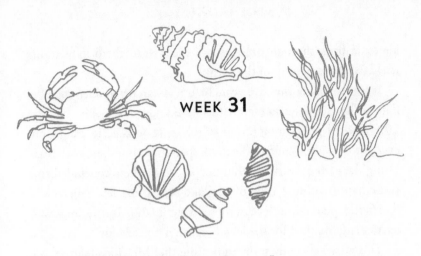

Walk Beside the Sea

IN THE FIRST PARAGRAPH OF *Moby-Dick*, the narrator—Ishmael—explains how the ocean acts on his mind and soul. Seeing "the watery part of the world," he says,

> is a way I have of driving off the spleen and regulating the circulation. Whenever I find myself growing dim about the mouth; whenever it is a damp drizzly November in my soul; whenever I find myself involuntarily pausing before coffin warehouses . . . I account it high time to get to sea as soon as I can.

The author, Herman Melville, knew instinctively that the sea lifts our mood, that somehow the ocean has the capacity to heal. Marine biologist Callum Roberts echoed Melville's words 165 years later: "People have a deep emotional connection to the sea. The oceans inspire, thrill and soothe us . . . Our relationship with the sea stretches back through time . . . all the way to the origins of life itself. We are creatures of the ocean."

It was to be another five years before researchers pulled together data to "prove" what so many of us have known all along. The year 2019 saw the publication of one of the most detailed investigations ever into the well-being effects of spending time beside the sea. Using data from nearly 26,000 people, researchers concluded that those living within a mile of England's coastline felt happier and had better mental health than those living inland. The findings were particularly marked for the lowest-earning households.

This wasn't the only study indicating that Melville's Ishmael was (in 1851) articulating something universally meaningful today. A report from New Zealand found the more people looked at the sea, the more relaxed, calm, and revitalized they felt. When it came to mood and well-being, the sea trumped everything, including greenery and trees. A 2016 study from the University of Exeter discovered that people living near the coast were "generally healthier and happier than those whose homes were inland," a finding corroborated by a study of elderly people in Ireland, where those with a sea view experienced less depression.

What is it about the sea that makes us feel so good? According to Professor Douglas Kenrick, constant overstimulation and mental clutter sends our brains "into overdrive," creating debilitating levels of stress. Our brains need recovery time, a chance to rest and replenish themselves. Or as Kenrick calls it, a period of "natural restoration." We do this most effectively when exposed to environments with a little bit of interest and novelty but also with a high degree of statistical predictability, keeping us engaged but simultaneously relaxed. Think of it as regularity without monotony, or familiarity without boredom, much like the river walk in Week 17 (p. 67). The sea might very well be the epitome of regularity without monotony: essentially unchanging, it also bewitches with its foaming waves, diving seabirds, and scattering light.

Others think the ocean's ebb and flow may contain the clue to its powerful mood-enhancing effects: namely that its pattern of continuous movement encourages our mind to move out of the vortex of its own thoughts.

There are other possible explanations, of course. According to the theory of biophilia, we automatically relax when we're close to sources of water and food, as if our brains carry ancient molecular memories of starvation and dehydration.

Some researchers think the omega-3 fatty acids found in oily fish and shellfish played a pivotal role in the development of the human brain: an innate, inarticulate knowledge that lures us back to a marine environment—as if we recognize the ocean as both home and a source of essential nourishment.

There's even a line of thought that seawater contains bacteria that enhances our immunity, creating in us an unconscious physiological pull to the ocean as we seek to replenish our microbiome.

Researchers have also investigated traits associated with the sea, speculating that the sounds of surf and breaking waves are deeply restorative, while reflections pique and engage our brain, and the fractal patterns of shells and waves soothe our frazzled minds.

But do we need up-to-the-minute science to entice us on a coastal walk? Sea cures were popular throughout the nineteenth century, millions of us spend our annual holiday beside the seaside, literature is awash in stories of the ocean, and over a third of the world's population chooses to live on the coast. Science simply confirms our often-compelling physiological need for the sea, reminding us to make time for a beach or clifftop walk.

So how often should we seek out the sea? Visiting twice weekly, or for two hours a week, gives us the best chance of good general and mental health, according to environmental psychologist Dr. Lewis Elliott.

TIPS

COASTAL WALKS ARE GENERALLY LESS crowded on wet days and in winter months.

Take binoculars: seabirds are often thrilling to watch.

Leave time for a dip: there's growing evidence that sea swimming reduces inflammation, possibly staving off dementia, not to mention reducing depression, anxiety, and mood swings. When Dr. Mark Harper studied sixty-one cold-water swimmers, he found significantly improved mood, which he attributed to lowered inflammation.

Sea walking (see Week 32: Walk in Water, p. 131) can be practiced year-round: just choose a stretch of safe, calm water.

Try walking barefoot: sand provides a natural form of resistance, strengthening leg muscles and core.

Can't get to the coast? Following a river is the next best thing (Week 17: Follow a River, p. 67).

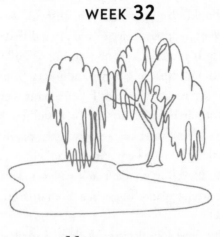

Walk in Water

IT WAS TWO-THIRTY IN THE afternoon, a week into the new year, when champion figure skater Nancy Kerrigan finished her practice session at an ice rink in Detroit. She was preparing for the 1994 U.S. Figure Skating Championships taking place a few days later. But that afternoon something happened that almost destroyed her career. As Kerrigan left the rink, she was struck savagely on her leg. Her assailant escaped by flinging himself through a glass door and leaping into a getaway car. Later it was discovered that he'd been hired by the husband of Kerrigan's opponent. Kerrigan was too injured to compete in the upcoming championships, but she was determined to compete in the Winter Olympics seven weeks later. This seemed ludicrously ambitious. And yet she astonished the world by winning a silver medal, missing gold by a hairsbreadth. How did she do this? By relearning her routine *in water*.

Walking in water liberates the body from the effects of gravity, providing a powerful low-impact cardio workout that builds strength in muscles not always engaged by land walking. Which is not to say we should give up swimming. Instead, we should view water as an enlivening opportunity to walk in a different way.

Water walking is ideal for anyone wanting to build muscle and burn calories without impacting bones and joints. The buoyancy of our bodies in water make it perfect for pregnant women, for the frail, for those with arthritis or osteoporosis, and for those recovering from injuries. When water bears our weight, we are free to move in ways that would otherwise be painful or difficult. After breaking multiple bones in a cycling accident, my sister-in-law (a chiropractor) regained her strength and fitness in a program of water walking she devised herself.

Several studies have found water walking beneficial for people with hip or knee osteoarthritis, chronic back pain, and spinal injuries. One study found twelve weeks of water walking helped patients with lumbar spinal stenosis recover their muscle and balance.

But water walking isn't only for the injured, frail, or pregnant. Because water is denser, it provides natural resistance twelve to fourteen times greater than the resistance we encounter on land, making water walking a superb way to build muscle and increase muscle tone. One study found water walking raised the heart rate more than land walking. Another found that unfit women reduced their blood pressure more dramatically after water walking than after normal walking.

Water walking is also excellent for developing balance, particularly if we practice in the sea, where sand or shingle shifting beneath our feet provides an additional challenge. And if that's not enough, water walking also increases our flexibility and range of motion: supported by the water, we can extend our limbs, safe in the knowledge that we won't be hurt if we topple over.

Lastly, there's evidence that water walking (like all walking) improves mood. People with fibromyalgia who tried water walking reported not only less stiffness and better cardiovascular health but a greater quality of life, with deeper sleep and less anxiety and depression—findings mirrored in studies of wild swimming, incidentally.

Gravity is greater the shallower the water, so to be entirely without gravity, you need to be submerged to the neck. However, thigh-deep water has been shown to provide a more intense workout than chest-deep water. The flip side is that chest-deep water uses less energy, enabling us to build greater endurance by walking for longer. To work your arms, you'll need chest-deep water with your arms swinging (or pushing) below the surface. Otherwise, opt for thigh-deep water or mix it up.

Getting started is easy. If you're walking in a pool, you need only a suit and a towel. If you're walking in the sea or a lake, consider wearing rubber sailing/water shoes or neoprene swim socks. Walk a length (40 to 80 feet is ideal), then return backward. Repeat. Next, sidestep a length. Repeat, swinging your arms as if you were walking on land. You'll feel the resistance immediately, but keep going.

Experiment with your stride length and (if it is possible and safe to do so) the water depth. Once you're comfortable, try lifting your knees higher and varying your speed. Introduce knee lifts, calf raises, jumps, walking lunges, or improvised dance moves. Indeed, many of the suggestions in this book are equally effective in water.

Incidentally, water walking is perfect for whiling away the hours supervising small children in water. No need to lie on the beach, your unblinking eye fixed on them. Just walk the water . . .

TIPS

KEEP YOUR ABDOMINAL MUSCLES ENGAGED, back straight, shoulders back, chin up, sight line directly in front—exactly the walking posture outlined in Week 2: Improve Your Gait (p. 10).

Not a strong swimmer? Wear a life jacket or use a buoyancy aid.

Avoid hot pools, and drink plenty of water—we don't always notice our thirst (or how much we're sweating) when immersed in water.

Consider wearing a wet suit if you're walking in the river or sea in the colder months.

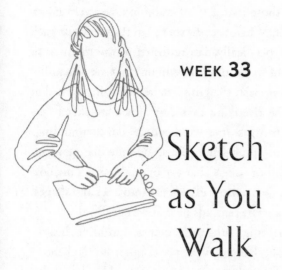

WEEK **33**

Sketch as You Walk

WHEN WE TAKE ENDLESS SNAPSHOTS on our phones, do we capture the moment or lose it? Last year, as I scrolled through hundreds of images, I sensed it was the latter. I often couldn't recall where I was or why I'd chosen to photograph a particular scene. The spots of time I had intended to preserve were effectively lost.

In the past, walkers and travelers often sketched and painted in the open air. Instead of returning with thousands of images that languished on a phone, they came home with a single sketchpad of salient scenes, which they lovingly shared and later bequeathed. It occurred to me that observing a scene as they had bore no resemblance to my (millions of) point-and-click snapshots.

So I set myself a challenge: to hike for two days without taking a photograph on my iPhone. Instead, I planned to sketch. A friend had told me that Picasso always traveled with a sketchbook, pencil, and eraser. I'm no Picasso, and I hadn't drawn since I gave up art classes at age fourteen. But I joined a drawing class and bought myself a sketchpad, pencil, and (most important) an eraser.

My sketches from those two days of walking aren't very good. But that's not the point. When I revisit them I'm thrown right back into that walk. More specifically, I'm returned to the moment of drawing . . . the smell of water mint, the sun on my neck, the milky jade-green water rushing past, the ginger-haired dog that sniffed at me as I perched on the riverbank that day. When we sketch, we *observe*. And when we truly observe, we encounter our surroundings quite differently—we are pulled into the scene, into the moment, with an intimacy and immediacy that excludes all else. Somehow we must transform that full sensory experience into lines and shapes, even color. Sketching a scene reminds us that we're fully alive.

But sketching also brings other advantages, including health-enhancing physiological changes. When a London hospital introduced an art program for patients, staff were stunned by the results. Patients making art "were significantly more likely . . . to have improved clinical outcomes, including better vital signs, diminished cortisol related to stress, and less medication needed to induce sleep."

A German study carried out a decade later provided a possible explanation. Researchers used brain-scanning techniques on two groups of retirees, one of which *looked* at works of art, while the other *made* art. The before-and-after scans showed that the creators of art had acquired greater spatial awareness than their nondrawing peers. But the researchers became most excited when they noticed "significant" changes to a particular brain region in the art-making group alone: the medial prefrontal cortex, known to play a vital role in psychological resilience and stress resistance. The researchers concluded that "visual art production has an impact on psychological resilience." No wonder other reviews have found creating art an excellent means of managing stress, burnout, depression, and anxiety.

Sketching is also good for our brain cells. An American study of 256 older adults found that drawing and painting were better at keeping the brain sharp than any other activity (including crafting, socializing, and computer games). The researchers wondered if making art could help develop new neural pathways, keeping our brain cells stimulated. In this study, those who started drawing and painting in midlife but persisted into old age saw the most benefits.

When we seek out scenes and objects to draw, our focus ceases to be on either ourselves or our destination. We're no longer racing to the top/the end/the lunch spot. We're no longer brooding. Instead, we're attending to little things along the way: a knuckled tree trunk bearded with blue lichen, the shape of a crane silhouetted against a dying sky, a church with a bewitchingly crooked steeple.

I sketch regularly now, enjoying the undivided attention it demands and the feelings of calm that accompany it. Drawing and painting help us look more closely, observe more thoroughly, so that even after the pad and pencil have been put away, our eyes are more attuned, better equipped to spot lines and colors, shapes and tones. More inclined to look outward than inward.

What's more, every instance of sketching is seared into my memory. No scrolling required . . .

TIPS

DON'T JUDGE YOUR DRAWINGS. They aren't intended for an exhibition, and no one need see them.

Experiment with different-size leads, charcoal, pen, and watercolor. Pocket-size watercolor sets are light and portable if you want to add color.

Look online for quick sketching tutorials or buy a how-to book.

Explore the styles of master sketchers. Then experiment—there are many different ways to draw.

Professional walking artists make full use of the weather and landscape, letting the rain mingle with their paint, pressing in grass and seed heads, using twigs instead of brushes, and painting with earth for example. Try doing the same.

Don't be restrained by time: a sketch need take only a few minutes, and you can always embellish it later. Some walking artists sketch on the fly, giving themselves mere seconds to capture a subject or scene—a sort of sight-snatching that any of us can emulate.

WEEK **34**

Walk Beneath a Full Moon

TWO DECADES AGO, I ARRIVED at a London hospital in the wrenching throes of childbirth. It was late in the evening and my contractions were growing steadily more painful. As I waited for a bed, I noticed the hospital seemed more charged than usual. I'd given birth to my first child in the same hospital and it hadn't seemed quite so . . . frantic. When my midwife finally arrived, she said something that left me slack-jawed and stupefied: "It's a full moon . . . everyone's giving birth!"

Engulfed by another contraction, I forgot her words. Until a decade later, when I began creeping out to walk at full moon. One night, walking through a moonlit field, I had a sudden flashback to the odd busyness of the maternity ward that evening. I went home and began trawling the internet. It didn't take long to find a study corroborating what my midwife had said. Researchers in the Japanese city of Kyoto compared the birth dates of 1,007 babies with the lunar cycle over a period of three decades. They found a significant increase in births during full-moon nights, concluding that "the gravitation of the Moon has an influence on the frequency of births."

During a full moon, gravitational pull increases because the moon and sun are pulling on the earth together. We know this explains ocean tides, but could it really have brought on my contractions? Well, for every report that finds a correlation, like the Kyoto study, there's another that finds no correlation whatsoever.

When it comes to human sleep patterns, the evidence is less controversial. A Swiss study published in the journal *Current Biology* and based on research done under "stringently controlled laboratory conditions" found the duration of deep sleep drops by 30 percent on full-moon nights. The same study also found that we typically take an additional five minutes to fall asleep, after which we sleep for twenty minutes *less* than on other nights. The researchers—who used EEGs (electroencephalogram) to record participants' sleep and saliva tests to measure their hormone levels—confirmed that levels of melatonin (the sleep hormone) fell and sleep quality was poorer around the time of a full moon. In conclusion, they claimed to "have evidence that the distance to the nearest full-moon phase significantly influences human sleep and evening melatonin levels." Their confidence was justified: at least three other reports have come to the same conclusions.

It's not merely our sleep that's affected by the lunar cycle. Several reports suggest that our behavior is also affected. Indeed, the word *lunatic* derives from the Latin word *luna*, moon. But once again, studies are erratic and inconsistent. A 2019 report explored homicides in Finland, linking their timings with the moon and finding that an incontrovertible "association exists between moon phases and homicides . . . homicides declined (by 15%) during the full moon." But in Florida quite a different story unfolded, with homicides and aggravated assaults clustering around full moons. Intriguingly, the Florida report also noted that "psychiatric emergencies decreased significantly" around new and full moons. Other reports found higher numbers of motorcycle accidents during full moons, and higher numbers of female suicides. On the other hand, a German study that matched up police records with lunar patterns found no whiff of correlation between homicides, assaults, or suicides and the full moon.

Clearly, links between our behavior and the full moon need further investigation. But does that mean disregarding the many studies that find a connection? Not so fast . . . Studies of animals show that behavior can and does change as a result of moonlight. It's now believed that circalunar clocks tick away inside many creatures, synchronizing their circadian clocks with a lunar-tidal clock. African dung beetles walk in straighter lines on moonlit nights. Certain sea creatures change their underwater positions according to the amount of night light. And Galápagos iguanas with very accurate circalunar clocks live longer than iguanas with less accurate clocks. Meanwhile, reports have linked the full moon with birthing patterns in European badgers and domestic cattle.

This could be the result of chance, of course. But why deny the possibility of lunar mysteries not yet elucidated? Indeed, many scientists are quite convinced that "the lunar effect" exists. It simply hasn't been completely untangled yet.

Besides, the strange, inexplicable findings of so many studies add to the eerie, enigmatic qualities of a moonlit walk. Beneath a clear sky and a full moon, the landscape shifts, so that it looks and feels quite different (see Week 46: Take a Night Walk, p. 190). Suddenly the idea that we too may be shifting and changing with the lunar cycle doesn't seem so outlandish.

The light of a full moon isn't—as one might expect—double that of a half-moon. Instead, it's ten times brighter, making the night sky too bright to stargaze but perfect for walking long distances, following a forest route, or spotting nocturnal wildlife.

More dramatic still are walks taken beneath supermoons, which typically occur twice a year on consecutive months. These are the biggest, brightest orbs of the year, with the moon at its fullest and at its closest point to Earth. Supermoon dates vary according to time zone, so check online, then choose a location, invite a friend or two—and hope for good weather.

Although supermoons are spectacularly bright, it's September's harvest moon that I love most. It rises early in the evening—usually around sunset—and often hangs just above the horizon, making it seem larger and brighter than other full moons. The harvest moon is also known for casting an ethereal orange glow. This frail amber hue exists because we're looking at the moon through a denser layer of Earth's atmosphere. Harvest moons keep their dramatic size, shape, and positioning for a couple of nights on either side, making this a thrilling time for a series of full-moon walks.

New moons mean far less light, making those nights particularly conducive to stargazing. New-moon nights may not have the dramatic, dazzling light of a full moon, but a slender crescent moon can be ethereally and delicately beautiful.

TIPS

CHECK ONLINE FOR THE EXACT dates and times of full moons, supermoons, and the harvest moon, remembering that they change every year and according to your location—and note these in a diary.

Follow the tips for a night walk (Week 46: Take a Night Walk, p. 190), but consider being more ambitious: a forest route where you can now walk without a head lamp, or a coastal route where moonbeams scattering on the ocean will delight and amaze.

Carefully chosen routes (avoiding shadowy hill descents, for example) can mean your path is illuminated all the way.

Spring full moons are excellent occasions to walk among rock pools, when the tide will be at its lowest (farthest out) and rock-pool creatures come to life, their fluorescence revealed with a UV flashlight (see Week 46, p. 190).

Don't forget the cold full moons of winter—there's nothing more exquisitely enigmatic than a full moon circled by clouds dense with ice crystals.

Pay attention to how you feel . . . Wilder? Less risk-averse? Less sleepy? Or exactly the same? Someday science might explain it.

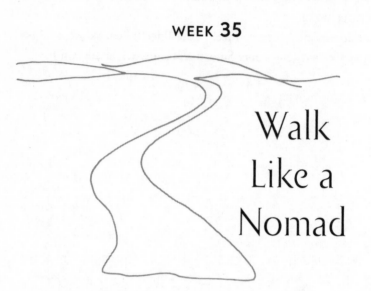

Walk Like a Nomad

IN 1980 A FRENCH RESEARCHER named Édouard Stiegler was working in Kabul when he noticed Afghan nomads arriving on foot at the local livestock market. Struck by their bright eyes and lively demeanor, he asked where they had come from. They told him they'd just arrived, that very day, from a 435-mile journey across deserts and over mountains. Stiegler was surprised. But it was the speed of their journey that left Stiegler speechless. The Afghan nomads had walked 435 miles in a mere twelve days. Stiegler began observing them, trying to understand how they walked 37 miles a day, and without any signs of fatigue. The answer, he deduced, was their breath-oriented mode of walking. The nomads practiced a conscious walking technique that involved synchronizing their breath with their (light and moderately paced) steps.

An inspired Stiegler returned to France and developed a hiking technique he named Afghan walking. His first book, *Régénération par la marche afghane*, was published a year later. Today Afghan walking is sometimes called breath-conscious hiking or even yogic hiking, and although it can be practiced by anyone, in any environment, it's particularly beneficial for endurance hikes. I make use of it when I'm hiking at altitude or taking part in long treks. But I also use it in my local London park when I need my mind emptied of its usual detritus, or when I want a few moments of inner calm. With its intense focus on rhythm and breathing, Afghan walking is almost meditative, making it adept at dispelling feelings of stress or anxiety.

The theory behind Afghan walking is simple. Efficient breathing allows our bodies to be properly oxygenated, enabling us to walk farther without feeling exhausted. Many of us don't breathe properly as we exercise, gulping rapidly at air through our mouths rather than matching our (full, nasal) inhalations to our stride. When we walk to the rhythm of our breath—or even breathe to the rhythm of our feet—we slow and lengthen our breathing. In combination with good posture (which Stiegler also noticed in the Afghan nomads), paced rhythmic breathing means that demanding mountain ascents and lengthy treks feel less tiring.

Afghan walking isn't complicated, but it benefits from a bit of practice. There are no hard-and-fast rules other than breathing entirely through our nose and in time to the tread of our feet. Once the basics have been mastered, we can experiment to find the timing that suits our stride, location, and fitness level. Stiegler suggests modifying our in-out breathing according to whether we're walking uphill or downhill, quickly or slowly, at sea level or at altitude, and according to our own levels of fitness.

Where to start? Stiegler recommends taking three inhalations through the nose, one with each step. On the fourth step we hold our breath. For the next three steps, we exhale (through the nose). On the subsequent step we neither inhale nor exhale, holding our lungs empty. Give it a try. You should have taken eight steps in total, one inhalation (in three parts/strides) and one exhalation (in three parts/strides) with a held breath after each. This 3–1:3–1 pattern is the basic breath-step technique of Afghan walking.

When walking uphill, you'll need to moderate your breathing. I prefer a 2:2 pattern for hill climbing: one two-part inhalation for each two steps, followed immediately by a two-part exhalation over two steps—and no held breaths. Find a rhythm that works with your own stride, pace, and landscape, ensuring step and breath are synchronized. Once mastered, Afghan walking feels splendidly liberating. There's something about walking to the rhythm of one's own breath, as if we can walk on and on, into the horizon and beyond.

Stiegler died shortly after his book was published, its many claims—which included better sleep, immunity, and cardiovascular health—never validated in his lifetime. This is changing—a group of researchers at the University of California recently wrote that mindful movement "may even outperform conventional physical exercise with regard to effects on quality of life, mood, and cognitive functioning." In his book *Breath: The New Science of a Lost Art*, James Nestor cites numerous studies linking correct breathing, like that of Stiegler's Afghan nomads, to lower blood pressure, improved immunity, denser bones, and better sleep (see Week 5: Breathe as You Walk, p. 22).

TIPS

YOUR BREATHING SHOULDN'T BE FORCED: take full, steady, slow breaths and synchronize with your steps, which shouldn't be too forced or fast, either. For more on breathing while walking, see Week 5 (p. 22).

Maintain good posture and walking gait (see Week 2: Improve

Your Gait, p. 10), so that your breath isn't too shallow. Unless you're hill climbing, your inhalations should reach down into your diaphragm.

Stiegler's second book, *Marcher respirer vivre*, suggests various breath-stride formulas, according to terrain, age, and fitness level, including a 6:6 pattern for the fittest among us.

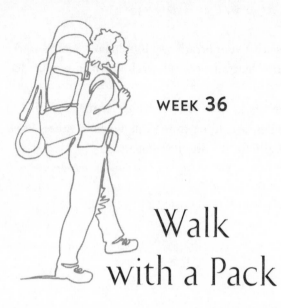

WEEK **36**

Walk
with a Pack

IN 1886, THE AMERICAN WRITER Alice Brown walked through England carrying her belongings on her back. "To walk is truly to live," she wrote in her memoir, claiming to have discovered how it feels "to fly like a pigeon, to live under water, to take root in the earth and grow." Brown believed that carrying her luggage (highly unusual for an educated woman in Victorian Britain) was an essential element in her journey of discovery, explaining that: "The feel of the pack is no burden but an added gift." Brown lived to the age of ninety-two—also highly unusual for a woman born in 1856.

Since then, millions of us—from Bill Bryson to Cheryl Strayed—have discovered the possession-less pleasures of backpacking. There's something endlessly liberating about strapping on a rucksack and walking for mile after mile. The feelings of independence, freedom, and autonomy sparked by long-distance walking are almost unrivaled. Finally we can cut ourselves loose from the cares and responsibilities of our everyday life. Besides, the world is full of thrilling landscapes and exhilarating trails, many so far off the beaten track that a backpack is obligatory.

As it happens, backpacking brings other lesser-known gifts: endurance and stamina. When we hike with a backpack, we transform a leisurely walk into a feat of endurance. In the military, brisk walking with a pack has its own name: rucking. The holy grail of endurance exercise, rucking is easier on the knees than jogging and, according to a study in the *British Journal of Sports Medicine*, free of the high injury rate of distance running. Rucking builds hip and postural stability, making us less susceptible to injury when we practice other sports. It provides a fantastically effective cardio workout: some studies suggest rucking burns through as many (if not more) calories than running. When we carry a backpack, our muscles work harder, keeping us and our load stable for hour after hour. And this reshapes and enlarges our heart. Screenings of endurance exercisers discovered their hearts to be different from the hearts of other people: longer, bigger, with more pliable left ventricles, enabling blood to be pumped with greater ease and efficiency. Sedentary people, or those exercising in short bursts, have smaller and stiffer hearts, making them more prone to heart disease and high blood pressure. Endurance exercisers often have very good metabolic health, meaning the rate at which they store fat and burn energy is perfectly balanced.

According to Professor Daniel Lieberman, human beings evolved as weight-bearing endurance walkers. He points out that nomadic tribespeople (particularly women, who do the lion's share of weight bearing) routinely carry 30 percent of their own body weight. Endurance, he explains, is something our bodies are uniquely suited to, the reason we have 5 to 10 million sweat glands and long, springy legs with elastic tendons. We evolved to walk and walk and walk—carrying babies, animal carcasses, water, and firewood. Perhaps this is why backpacking feels so curiously right, as if we're tapping into a deeply held molecular memory.

Walking with a pack also strengthens the muscles running from our spine through our buttocks and the backs of our legs, known as the posterior chain—a skein of muscles left languishing by our sedentary lifestyle but imperative for bending, jumping, and standing up, and vital for good posture. When we walk with weight on our back, our chest opens (enabling us to breathe with greater ease and efficacy), our core is activated, and our posterior chain is put to work.

As if all this isn't enough, early research also indicates that walking while bearing weight can improve—and even restore—the ability to think. Experiments in which rats climbed ladders with bags of pellets attached to their bodies revealed their postworkout brains to be teeming with new enzymes and neurons, so that even rodents with mild dementia effectively went into remission, their cognitive abilities "effectively restored."

Contented backpacking requires a little planning and preparation. Build your strength and endurance with regular daily walks, wearing a partially filled backpack if you want. Better still, leave the car at home and do your weekly shopping on foot with a backpack. Back-strengthening exercises can help. Fitness coach to the military Stew Smith recommends preparing with a program of dead lifts, squats, and lunges with hand weights. Try day and weekend hikes before embarking on a longer trek, so that your body adjusts gradually to the full weight of a rucksack.

Stay motivated by planning a distance hike, pinning a picture of it to your wall or making it your screen saver. Numerous new trails have been created in the last decade, and hundreds of ancient trails restored. A plethora of apps have made it possible to create and share trails or to walk in the footsteps of earlier walkers. Arguably, there's never been a better time to pick up a pack and walk. Moreover, routes like this are perfect for women of all ages. According to Dr. Lisa Mosconi, "Low-to-moderate intensity exercise optimizes metabolic performance in women, especially when sustained over time." There's more on this subject in Week 40: Walk Like a Pilgrim (p. 165).

TIPS

INVEST IN THE RIGHT BACKPACK. It should have a padded back, a padded hip belt, and padded shoulder straps.

Wear it correctly: always use the hip belt and the chest strap. These help transfer the weight from your back and shoulders, distributing it across your entire upper body.

Tighten the straps so that the pack sits snugly against your body. Your waist straps should be as tight as possible without being uncomfortable.

If the pack is hitting your backside, it's too low. If it's above your head, it's too high.

When packing, put the heavier things closer to the back (where it meets your spine) and the lighter things closer to the outer edges. Lieberman suggests putting the heavier items toward the top and leaning slightly forward in order to save energy as you hoist the pack on and off.

Bend at the knees when lifting your pack, and never carry it with one strap.

Don't hunch, open your chest—imagine an ice cube dropped down your back.

Find an appropriate pace: neither too fast nor too slow. Go too fast and you'll exhaust or injure yourself. Go too slow and your shoulders will ache from the weight of the pack.

Hike only in boots you know and love.

Walking with poles will add to your upper body workout. According to Martin Christie, founder of Nordic Walking UK, using poles (either trekking or Nordic) means we engage 90 percent of our muscles.

Poles also help with balance—important when backpacking, as a large pack makes you less stable. Small steps also help with balance, so shorten your stride when going downhill and over uneven terrain.

Warming up, cooling down, and stretching are vital when rucking, according to seasoned rucker Lieutenant Captain Liam O'Kelly. Stretching while the muscles are warmed from walking also improves flexibility.

Stay well hydrated, drinking water before, during, and after a long ruck.

Take a friend: studies show we perceive distances as shorter and less daunting when we have a friend with us. But don't worry if you're walking solo: the same studies show that merely imagining a friend at your side has the same effect.

WEEK 37

Take a
Foraging Walk

IN SEPTEMBER 1943, A NOT-YET-KNOWN Patience Gray took her children to live in a remote run-down cottage hidden deep in a Sussex woodland. The nearest shop was a four-mile round trip, which they walked twice a week. Meanwhile, Gray began collecting mushrooms, taking them home to identify and cook, and sparking an insatiable appetite for foraging. She foraged for the rest of her life, most famously in France, Spain, Greece, and Italy, where she wandered for days collecting edible plants. The result was her cult classic, *Honey from a Weed*.

A foraging walk immerses us in nature in a way no other walk can. We find ourselves, literally, in the thorny heart of a blackberry bush, the smell of berries in our nose, the stain of juice on our skin, the song of an envious bird in our ear. This is nature at its most visceral and delicious. Foraging, maintained Gray, allows us to fully "experience the human–plant relation."

Foraging walks are also a chance to amble for hours, collecting (and often eating) as we go, accompanied by friends, grandparents, and children. Anyone can forage, but children have a natural affinity for it. Gray gleaned much of her foraging knowledge from "children [who] wandered about in February and March . . . in search of weeds." One of her best "weed lessons" came from a seven-year-old girl who knew how to cook and eat every wild plant in her father's vineyard.

Anthropologists studying hunter-gatherers in Tanzania found children over the age of five to be particularly avid foragers with a sharp eye for fruit, birds, tubers, honey, and small game. My twelve-year-old daughter has a nose so attuned to sniffing out wild truffles, she almost put a trained truffle hound out of business. Hardly surprising, then, that evolutionary psychologists believe our urge to forage runs deep in our blood, encoded somehow in our DNA.

Where we live determines what we can forage for. On the Greek island of Naxos, Gray foraged for wild chicory and endive, milk thistle, and marigolds. In Italy, she found wild asparagus and wild beets. In England, she collected field mushrooms, nettles, and sorrel. While I was growing up on the Welsh coast, my family foraged for crabs, puffballs, and blackberries. In the last two decades I've forage-walked for bilberries, wild raspberries, and cloudberries (Norway); walnuts (Spain); samphire (Norfolk); mussels (Ireland); truffles (Sussex); chestnuts (London); and rose hips, dandelion leaves, wild garlic, elderflowers, nettles, water mint, and blackberries (pretty much everywhere). There's nothing more gratifying than returning home weighed down with fresh, free produce—all the more so when we know that many foraged goodies are so-called superfoods, rich in vitamins, minerals, and phytonutrients.

A list of the top eleven superfoods recently published in Everyday Health—and based on an original list from the U.S. National Institutes of Health (NIH)—included seven foods readily available in the wild: berries, seafood, garlic, mushrooms, leafy greens, nuts, and seeds.

The ubiquitous blackberry is packed with antioxidants and vitamins C, A, and K. Studies of rats fed blackberries found they had improved balance and coordination, as well as "significantly greater short-term memory." The extraordinary properties of mushrooms are well known, and mycotherapy—the medicinal use of mushrooms—is being investigated as a breast cancer treatment. Dandelion leaves are rich in iron, calcium, potassium, and magnesium as well as multiple vitamins (A, C, K, E, and B). Early studies suggest nettle tops can reduce levels of inflammation, blood sugar, and blood pressure. The leaves of wild garlic (sometimes called ransoms) are particularly effective at reducing blood pressure, according to one study, but like all garlic are antifungal and antibacterial, as well as rich in phytochemicals. Nuts and seeds are excellent sources of protein, antioxidants, and fiber, with a recent study from Loma Linda University suggesting that a daily handful of nuts significantly lowers cholesterol.

I typically forage-walk in spring and in autumn. In spring I collect dandelion leaves and nettle tops (April), wild garlic and elderflowers (May/June). And in autumn, crab apples, blackberries, sloes, rose hips, and damsons (August/September) and truffles, mushrooms, and nuts (September/October). You can work out your own foraging calendar according to where you live and what you and your family and friends like to eat, drink, preserve, or cook.

A good foraging guide is essential—consider it an investment. Seek out guides that specialize in the terrain or state you intend to forage from. Many will contain recipes for your safely foraged ingredients, including pestos, preserves, liqueurs, salads, and syrups.

TIPS

NEVER EAT ANYTHING YOU'RE UNSURE OF. Guided foraging expeditions are an excellent way of discovering what's safe to eat in your area.

Pick sustainably, don't take more than you need, don't dig up protected plants, and avoid private land.

Foraging is subject to complicated legislation so make sure you know the laws for the area in which you're foraging. Some states prohibit all foraging on state land, while others take a more relaxed approach. Foraging on private property is always against the law.

Avoid foraging in areas of sewage, pollution, dogs, and pesticides/herbicides. Wash your weeds well.

Take plenty of containers or walk like a genuine Mediterranean forager in a homemade apron with three pockets (one for bitter greens, one for sweet greens, and the last for roots and fungi, apparently).

Worried about the temptations of over-snacking? No need. Researchers at a British university found that a 15-minute walk curbed our cravings for snacking (on chocolate). But when the snack on offer is a blackberry, why worry?

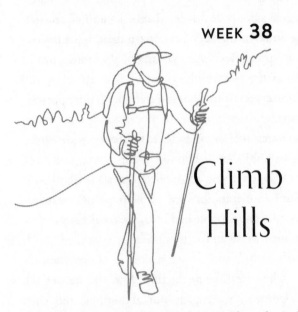

Climb Hills

IT WAS A MILD DAY in April 1336 when the Italian poet Petrarch set off to climb Mont Ventoux in the south of France. He was accompanied by his brother, who had no hesitation in taking the most direct path "straight up the ridge." Petrarch, however, hunted out obscure winding paths that meant he could avoid steep ascents altogether. "I did not mind going further if only the path were less steep," he wrote in his account. Unfortunately, several of the routes he pursued went down rather than up, so that all he did was "increase the distance and difficulty." As his brother lay resting at the summit, Petrarch cursed himself for "trying to avoid the exertion of the ascent."

Six hundred years later the writer Nan Shepherd (a woman without a shred of Petrarch's self-proclaimed laziness) declared her love of "toiling" uphill. For her, the exertion of the ascent was precisely the point. She recognized that the thrilling sense of well-being she experienced in the hills was a direct result of the sustained rhythm of movement in a long climb.

Shepherd has science on her side. Toiling uphill—however slowly—works the body as intensely as running does, boosting our heart rate, burning up calories, and sparking the famous flush of endorphins known as the runner's high. But unlike running, hill climbing neither impacts our joints nor interferes with our appreciation of the landscape.

Hill walking activates different muscles from those we use on flat land. When we hike uphill, our abdominal, hip, glute, and back muscles come into play, engaging to stabilize our skeleton. This is because, as we climb, we lean forward to help propel ourselves upward. According to a paper published in the journal *Gait & Posture*, the glutes, hamstrings, and calf muscles are worked much harder when we walk uphill. Indeed, we make use of every muscle in our lower body when we hike an incline. And the steeper the climb, the more vigorously we engage our abdominal and back muscles—in order to keep us upright.

As our arms swing, our body twists slightly, meaning the muscles on either side of our waist (the obliques) are also put to work. All this balancing and stabilizing of our skeleton means hill walking is superb exercise for the core, particularly if we're walking across varied terrain where our body must rebalance with every step. An uphill toil connects us, more than any other walk, with our own pumping heart.

Interestingly, uphill and downhill walking use different muscles—with different effects on our body. When we walk uphill, our muscles shorten (a concentric contraction). But when we walk downhill, our body works against the pull of gravity and so our muscles lengthen (an eccentric contraction). When scientists from the Austrian Vorarlberg Institute compared the blood sugar, cholesterol, and triglyceride levels of uphill versus downhill walkers, they found that, although both groups reduced their LDL ("bad") cholesterol, only uphill walkers reduced their triglycerides (fats linked to heart disease and strokes). But what most baffled the researchers was the unexpected impact of downhill walking: it was twice as effective at improving glucose tolerance and removing blood sugars. The researchers concluded that downhill walking might be an excellent option for diabetics or for older people new to exercise. For the rest of us, this is a reminder to walk both up and down the hill.

There's another reason we should add hill walking to our repertoire. A recent study found those who mixed their regular walking with something brisker became more efficient walkers. How does this work? We become less efficient walkers as we age, requiring more and more oxygen to walk at the same pace as a younger person—and tiring more easily as a result. But a study conducted by Professor Justus Ortega found that efficient walkers in old age were far more likely to mix up their exercise by including something more intense than moderate walking (like running or cycling . . . or hill walking) once or twice a week. Professor Ortega told *The New York Times* that more demanding exertions boosted the health and function of mitochondria (the powerhouses of our cells) in ways that gentler walking did not. The better our mitochondria, the more efficient our movement, and hence the less tired we are when we walk. Hill walking is the apotheosis of mixed-up movement, with its bursts of climbing, descending, and walking on the flat.

Of course, hill walking brings numerous other joys. Some of us appreciate the thinner air of high elevations (see also Week 23: Walk at Altitude, p. 92), including Nan Shepherd, who believed that as the air became rarer and more stimulating, she felt lighter and walked with less effort. Sweeping views shift our eyes into panorama mode (see Week 8: Walk with Vista Vision, p. 33). Hills give us silence, scent, and solitude (see Weeks 22, 39, and 15). But more than anything, hill climbing gives us a profound sense of satisfaction, of physical accomplishment. We are, quite literally, on top of the world. The pioneering mountain climber Mary Mummery expressed it perfectly when, in 1887, she reached the famously challenging Alpine summit of Täschhorn in a thunderstorm: "True it was late; true we were cold, hungry and tired; true we were sinking into the snow above our knees; but the *Teufelsgrat* [ridge] was ours and we cared little for these minor evils."

TIPS

USE WALKING POLES. NOT ONLY do poles provide a full-body workout, enabling the shoulders and arms to be worked (and to take some of the weight), but using poles also delays feelings of tiredness on long ascents, according to a study published in the *European Journal of Applied Physiology*. On descents, poles reduce the weight on knee and hip joints. Shorten your poles going uphill and lengthen them going downhill.

Find a slow, steady rhythm and make use of Afghan breathing (see Week 35: Walk Like a Nomad, p. 144).

Shorten your stride: smaller steps are better for both uphill and downhill. (Descending puts twice as much pressure on knee joints as walking on the flat.)

Make sure your walking boots fit well and have good ankle support. Consider adding extra cushioning (like an insole or extra-thick sock) to take some of the additional impact generated by going downhill.

Hill climbing isn't an easy alternative to hill running: walking a steep gradient builds stronger calf muscles than running a steep gradient, explaining why some experts recommend that runners include uphill walking in their training programs.

Take a friend: when we hike with a pal, hills appear less steep, according to one study.

Walking uphill can aggravate lower back pain. Start slowly and build up speed and duration as your back muscles strengthen.

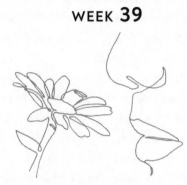

Walk with Your Nose

IN AN UNPUBLISHED FRAGMENT FOUND after her death, the writer and marine biologist Rachel Carson wrote that whenever she thought of the warblers on her island walks, the recollection was accompanied by a great rush of perfume: "The scent of all the heady aromatic bitter-sweet fragrances compounded of pine and spruce and bayberry, warmed by the sun through the hours of a July day." Smell has a genius for doing this, for returning us instantly to a time and place, making our nose a supremely satisfying walking companion.

We don't process smell in the way we process our other senses. Instead of being filtered through a brain part called the thalamus— where sensations are registered and processed—smell travels directly to our primary olfactory cortex, which lies deep within our brain. Olfaction—our sense of smell—is the most primitive of our five senses. Millennia back, it was our capacity to smell that helped us find food and avoid danger. Today, our screen-based lives have left our sense of smell languishing. And yet our nose is astonishingly sophisticated, a sort of chemical sensor device containing 350 odor-receptor genes developed over millions of years and capable of detecting the lightest and subtlest of smells. Walking enables us to reconnect with our sense of smell, a sense with almost improbable implications for our body and brain.

In the last few decades, researchers investigating the effects of inhaling essential oils have reported surprising results. Aromatic compounds found in pine, rosemary, lavender, and tens of other plants have been linked to the alleviation of pain and anxiety; the suppression of some cancer tumors; reduced inflammation; improved sleep; enhanced mood; and better focus, attention, and memory.

Perhaps the results shouldn't surprise us. After all, essential oils have been used for centuries. The Egyptians were blending aniseed, cedar, and myrrh into ointments as far back as 4500 BCE. A few centuries later, Chinese and Indian healers had listed over 700 aroma therapeutic plants, including cinnamon, ginger, and sandal-wood. The Greeks followed suit, documenting their use of thyme, saffron, lavender, and peppermint. Today these oils are widely used by the pharmaceutical industry, their biochemical properties having proven to be anti-inflammatory, antimicrobial, antiviral, antiseptic, anticarcinogenic, and antifungal.

The intranasal pathway is now fully recognized as an entry route to the brain, via the lungs and blood. Scent molecules cross the blood-brain barrier to interact with our central nervous system, causing immediate physiological changes, from alterations to our blood pressure and muscle tension, to shifts in our pulse rate and brain activity.

Pine needle oil has been found to arrest the proliferation of cancer cells, with one study suggesting that oil extracted from the needles of Scots pine could help suppress tumors in some forms of breast cancer. Numerous studies on both rodents and people have found that inhaling rosemary oil improves memory, sharpens focus, reduces inflammation, and alleviates pain.

Other studies suggest that "lavender inhalation can significantly reduce anxiety levels" and improve feelings of relaxation. In fact lavender is the most heavily researched oil, and findings of its efficacy—which also include deeper sleep and improved concentration—are incontrovertible. In hospital patients, the smell of peppermint oil has successfully curbed nausea and vomiting. When inhaled, sage oil dramatically slows the pulse rates of anxious patients. Among those with Alzheimer's, oil of lemon balm has improved memory and mood.

Researchers from Sussex University found that a sniff of lemon oil (already known to increase the production of white blood cells and to strengthen immunity) changes how we *feel* about our bodies, making us feel *thinner and lighter*. In other words, certain smells also have the power to work on our emotions.

Many of these densely perfumed plants and herbs grow abundantly in the wilds. Hiking the coast near Marseille recently, I was accompanied by an intoxicating cloud of lavender, sage, thyme, and rosemary. Later, while I was walking in the Spanish Sierra Nevada, my scented companions included wild basil and fennel. Both hikes are etched brightly in my memory, something I attribute to the dazzling aromatic air and the proven links between certain oils and memory.

Plants are at their most intensely aromatic in heat or after rain (ideally in heat following a downpour!), but we can enjoy their scents by rubbing their leaves, berries, or petals between our fingers as we walk, or by snapping a dead twig (in the case of juniper, for example) and inhaling directly from it. Amazingly, our scent cells are replaced every one to two months. Why waste them?

TIPS

SEEK OUT AREAS RICH IN aromatic plant life: pine forests, blue-bell woods, the damp minty banks of streams and rivers, the herb-strewn tracks of Mediterranean hills. In cities, look for wooded parks and formal rose or herb gardens.

Walk slowly, periodically closing your eyes and putting your hands over your ears to help direct attention back to your odor-receptor cells.

Slowly exhale immediately after breathing in an aroma: on its return voyage past our olfactory sensors, the scent amplifies.

If smelling directly from a flower, use the perfumer's technique of taking a series of short, shallow sniffs (to flood our olfactory receptors).

Warmer days are best—many flowers release greater profusions of scent on days when insects are most abundant.

For a city smell walk, try Week 11: Take a City Smell Walk (p. 44).

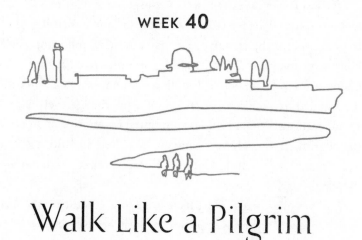

Walk Like a Pilgrim

ON THE FIRST DAY OF 1953, the woman later known as Peace Pilgrim left her home and began walking. She wore a navy tunic emblazoned with the words *25,000 miles on foot for peace.* In her pack she had a single change of clothes, a toothbrush, and a comb, but no money. Indeed, Peace Pilgrim never used or carried money again. Nor did she ever resume a normal life. Instead, she walked: twenty-five miles a day through America, Canada, Mexico; through the night; through heat, snow, and storms. Her pilgrimage continued for the remaining twenty-eight years of her life. Where did she find the energy, the stamina, the courage? "God," she explained, attributing her remarkable health to her deep spirituality.

Pilgrimage as a self-imposed, spiritual journey on foot has existed for centuries. As far back as the year 1300, 3,000 pilgrims arrived in Rome every day. In Japan, written accounts of pilgrimage—the only time many women left their homes—date back to the Heian period (794 to 1185). The first Muslim pilgrimage to Mecca (known as the Hajj) took place in the year 628.

The last few decades have seen a resurgence of pilgrims—walkers seeking spiritual rejuvenation, wanting to join something greater than themselves by stepping out, day after day, following ancient pilgrimage routes. In 2019, 350,000 pilgrims arrived at Santiago de Compostela in Spain, while 2 million went on the Hajj. Three hundred and thirty million people go on a pilgrimage every year. In recent years, new organizations committed to restoring and promoting pilgrimage routes have sprung up, including the British Pilgrimage Trust, Italy's South Cultural Routes project, and Norway's National Pilgrim Centre.

And yet pilgrimages don't have to be long distances. The medieval pilgrim Margery Kempe was a great believer in the micropilgrimage—distances of two miles or less to the nearest holy site. According to the British Pilgrimage Trust, it's not about the *how long*, but about the *how*.

So what makes a pilgrimage different from a walk? Firstly, a pilgrimage requires a *destination with meaning*. In the past this was typically a holy place, but today it might be an ancient tree, the house of an admired painter or architect, somewhere that holds special memories for us, or the site of a rare orchid. Secondly, a pilgrimage requires an *intention*. This can be as simple as plotting out our day's work or emptying our mind before bed. Alternatively, it can be more reflective, more challenging: a problem we want help with or something to want to give thanks for.

Nor does a pilgrimage have to follow a traditional pilgrim route. My most significant *route of remembrance* is along the beach where my father strolled on the last day of his life. "With pilgrimage you literally walk a physical path, have a clear goal—your destination—and a means of reaching it: walking. The simplicity . . . may be the secret to finding inner-direction," Dr. Guy Hayward of the British Pilgrimage Trust told *The Guardian* newspaper.

Simplicity is all well and good. But are we more likely to experience some sort of spiritual transcendence on a genuine, authentic pilgrimage? Nancy Frey, an expert on the pilgrimage to Santiago de Compostela, certainly believes so: "When pilgrims begin to walk several things . . . happen . . . they develop a changing sense of time, a heightening of the senses, and a new awareness of their bodies and the landscape." During her observations, Frey noticed that pilgrims connected deeply with the environment around them, developing a "strong sense of the here and now."

Researchers involved in a Yale-Columbia study found that spiritual experience involves "pronounced shifts in perception [that] buffer the effects of stress," confirming earlier reports linking spiritual experience to greater resilience.

Numerous studies during recent years have investigated the place of spirituality and faith in our health, both physical and mental. Several found that a sense of the spiritual promoted higher levels of life satisfaction and well-being, a clearer sense of purpose and meaning, greater hope and optimism, as well as lower levels of depression and anxiety. More enigmatically, some reports indicated a correlation between spiritual practice and longevity. Associate Professor Marino Bruce, author of one such report, explained how feeling that:

> you're not in the world alone, that you're part of a power larger than oneself, can give one confidence to deal with the issues of life. Biologically, if that reduces stress, then that means you're less likely to have high blood pressure or diabetes or things that can increase mortality.

Or perhaps our spiritual experiences are the result of a complicated cocktail of neurochemicals. A 2008 study linked spiritual experience to raised levels of multiple neurochemicals, including dopamine, melatonin, endorphins, and the happiness transmitter, serotonin. Accepting that our out-of-body experiences (for want of a better term) either trigger or are triggered by physiological factors doesn't diminish them. Rather, it illuminates them.

Whatever our beliefs, a pilgrimage, in which we are "companioned" by the thousands who previously walked our route and by the pilgrims currently walking beside us, may provide a collective sense of solace that other walks don't.

Although pilgrimages can be short, the traditional pilgrim routes typically require days (and days!) of steady walking, otherwise known as stamina and endurance. According to Lisa Mosconi in her book *The XX Brain*, this is exactly the sort of movement that women excel at and benefit from. Women possess a preponderance of "Type 1 muscle fibers . . . sugar burning estrogen and . . . greater capillary density," she explains. This powerful combination means we use glucose with particular efficiency. It also helps our blood circulate, for hour after hour, through our muscle tissue. Women are better at endurance, declares Mosconi, adding that "most women need to exercise for longer periods at lower intensity to boost metabolism and optimize aerobic fitness." Which is exactly what happens when we walk and walk . . .

TIPS

CONSIDER ENDING YOUR WALK AT a place of worship. The British Pilgrimage Trust suggests timing your finish to coincide with an evening church service.

Pilgrimage expert Clare Gogerty, in her 2019 book *Beyond the Footpath*, recommends keeping a pilgrimage journal, learning the names of the flora and fauna along your route, and turning off your phone.

Walking a pilgrim route is an excellent option for those wanting to walk alone, but with the chance of company. Pilgrims on routes like the Camino de Santiago often forge lifelong friendships. See Week 15: Walk Alone (p. 59) and Week 43: Walk with Others (p. 177).

The literature of pilgrimage is alive and kicking. For inspiration, try Guy Stagg's *The Crossway*, Justin Butcher's *Walking to Jerusalem*, or GirlTrek's online account of walking in the footsteps of Harriet Tubman.

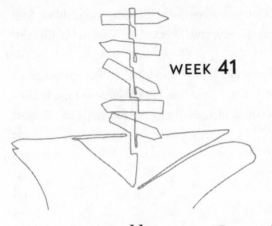

WEEK **41**

Walk to Get Lost

IN 1955, THE FRENCH THEORIST Guy Debord coined the terms *psychogeography* and *le dérive* (the drift) to describe urban walks made solely to explore our psychological response to the landscape. The antithesis of Week 25's Walk with Purpose (p. 101) or Week 40's Walk Like a Pilgrim (p. 165), *le dérive* requires us to get lost, to stroll without intention or agenda, to embrace the forgotten corners of a city.

I often drift in my home city of London—not because I'm a psychogeographer but because I like getting lost. I like the way it jolts me awake, as if a double espresso has been poured directly into my head and given a good stir. When we're lost, we're exposed to new landscapes and landmarks—forcing our brain to sit up and take note, to engage with our surroundings. The brain loves novelty. Confronted with something new or different, our brains immediately build new neural pathways, improving our memory and our capacity for learning in the process.

Neuroscientists have discovered that the brain regions known as the substantia nigra and the ventral tegmental area (crucial for learning and memory) are activated by new images, particularly when those images are positive or pleasing. This combination of pleasure and novelty triggers the creation of new neurons while simultaneously rewarding us with a shot of dopamine.

When we're lost (or think we're lost), our brain scrambles to protect us, making us interact with the landscape with renewed vigor. This is the reverse of what happens when we're guided by Google Maps. Blindly following a little red dot, we fail to notice what's above, below, or behind us. With our landscapes tamed and translated, we miss the richness around us—from the tiny architectural flourishes historically used by builders to personalize their work, to the glimmer of green as new leaves unfurl. But we also lose the startling thrill of stumbling into the unknown, of encountering somewhere unexpected, somewhere utterly novel.

When we're lost, we're also forced to develop our wayfinding skills (the skills set in motion by Week 24's Walk with a Map, p. 96). This is particularly important for women, who are still perceived to be less adept at orienting themselves in space. Spatial skills, says anthropologist Elizabeth Cashdan, "are the largest cognitive sex difference known." Cashdan—who has investigated spatial skills in cultures around the world as well as in other species—says this has nothing to do with the female brain and everything to do with cultural conditioning and female confidence. While males historically traveled farther afield and into less familiar territory in their hunt for food and mates, females were encouraged to stay closer to home. Undernourished, their navigational skills languished and their place and grid cells atrophied. Studies now link wider areas of travel, regardless of one's sex, with greater spatial cognition. In other words, the more time we spend map-less, negotiating unfamiliar terrain, the better our spatial understanding.

More significantly, our new awareness of the brain's plasticity means that any of us can rewire our brains to be spatially competent. According to Professor Sheryl Sorby, we can do this at any age and with as little as fifteen hours of training.

Spatial cognition isn't just an issue of gender. It's also an issue of *age*. From our teenage years on, our ability to orient ourselves in space declines. Like any cognitive skill, the ability to wayfind needs practice. Getting lost on foot is an excellent way of improving our spatial orientation, forcing our brain to use all the resources at its disposal.

Getting-lost walks are, paradoxically, most effective when they're planned. Losing oneself can quickly tip from exciting to terrifying—if we find ourselves somewhere dark and dangerous or if we have no access to food and water, for example.

TIPS

WALKING TO GET LOST IS an excellent way of unraveling a new city, but always carry a map.

Unexplored areas often lie on our doorstep, or within a short bus or train ride. To fully enjoy getting lost, choose an area that is safe and walkable.

Start in the morning: going into the unknown is more unsettling when the light fades.

Take a map, a compass, a phone (for emergencies only) and a charger or spare battery, a water bottle, and snacks.

Choose the right companions. (Getting lost is not for everyone.) Guy Debord recommends drifting in groups of two or three.

Even better, go alone. In his book, *Wayfinding: The Art and Science of How We Find and Lose Our Way*, Michael Bond urges us to explore on our own, because only when we are completely alone do we make full, un-delegated use of our locational skills.

A Debord-style *dérive* can last from a few minutes to several days, with an "average duration" of one day. To learn more, read Debord's *Theory of the Dérive*, which can be found online.

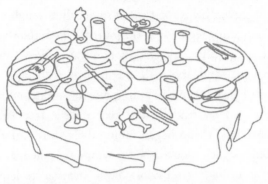

Walk After Eating

WHY DO SO MANY OF us think exercising after a large meal is detrimental to our health? I grew up convinced—thanks to my grandmother—that digestion works best if we sit and rest after eating. Exercise, she warned me, meant cramps, indigestion, and worse. For decades I barely moved after a meal. The larger the meal, the less I moved. Indeed, I was so in thrall to my grandmother's advice that I spent large chunks of my years as a mother trying to persuade my unruly children to sit still after meals. Lingering over a long meal, I explained, was essential for our health.

Only the most rigorous of science has, after forty-odd years, managed to shake off the no-movement-after-a-meal myth. It turns out that the reverse is true: gentle exercise after a meal has numerous benefits, from helping prevent constipation to lowering blood glucose levels. The perfect gentle exercise is of course walking. Or strolling. Or sauntering.

What's more, the bigger the meal, the greater our body's need for a postprandial walk. The good news (for those averse to long walks) is that a ten-minute stroll is all it takes to lower the blood glucose spikes that can be triggered by overeating.

When it comes to digestion, it appears that the combination of exercise and gravity helps food travel smoothly through our digestive systems. A study reported in the journal *Gut* found that "transit time was dramatically accelerated by moderate exercise," while defecation frequency and stool weight remained unchanged. In other words, exercise helps keep everything moving, reducing our risk of constipation. A later study found that middle-aged sufferers of chronic constipation who began taking daily thirty-minute walks reduced many of their blocked-bowel symptoms (ahem . . . reduced time spent "straining," softer stools, fewer "incomplete defecations") as well as speeding up "total colonic transit time."

It's not only our digestion that responds favorably to walking after eating. A fascinating 2016 study found that walking after a meal was better for regulating our blood sugar levels than walks taken at any other time of day. In this study, researchers wanted to understand whether people with type 2 diabetes were better off taking a ten-minute stroll after a main meal or taking a single thirty-minute walk. The researchers found that shorter, more frequent walks (particularly when taken after eating) lead to lower blood glucose levels than a single daily half-hour walk. Interestingly, the most dramatic effects were found when participants took an after-dinner walk. These walks resulted in blood glucose levels falling 22 percent further than the levels in people taking a single daily walk, emboldening the researchers (at New Zealand's University of Otago) to suggest that after-eating walks could reduce the need for insulin injections. A more recent meta-study confirmed these findings, with the authors agreeing that "exercise performed post-meal regardless of time of day had a beneficial impact on postprandial glycemia" (meaning blood glucose levels).

We don't need to be diabetic to reap the advantages of a post-meal saunter. Even the blood glucose levels of nondiabetics can spike after a heavy meal. Many of us typically eat more carbohydrates in the evening, often loading up on pasta, pizza, potatoes, rice, or bread. Moreover, as darkness falls, we're more inclined to slouch on the sofa (or retire to bed). Instead, we should be taking a short stroll, whatever the weather. The very last thing we should be doing is reaching for the remote control or—worse still—curling up under the duvet.

In the same way that walking after a meal speeds up the transit of waste through the gut, so it speeds up the passage of nutrients (from our recently gobbled meal), delivering vital biochemicals, vitamins, and minerals efficiently to their appropriate destination. Think of movement after eating as a little like drizzling oil into a rusty lock, easing food—and its nutrients—through our bodies.

When I started taking after-dinner strolls (sometimes with a friend or daughter, sometimes with the husband, often on my own), I also discovered some additional benefits. Firstly, I drank less wine. There wasn't much point topping up my glass when I was going out. Secondly, I was less inclined to keep picking at food on the table—knowing I was about to walk stopped my natural tendency to pick at leftovers. Thirdly, my stroll reinvigorated me, and I returned home better able to concentrate and more inclined to read than to flop on the sofa. Lastly, I often slept better. Perhaps because the evening gloom had helped trigger the production of melatonin (for more on light, dark, and our circadian clock, see Week 10: Walk Within an Hour of Waking, p. 40), or because my paced breathing had calmed me (see Week 51: Walking as Meditation, p. 211).

Nor is there any need to feel guilty about the (short) duration of your evening walk. Ten minutes is fine, as proposed by the Otago researchers. But additional studies also suggest that three ten-minute walks may be more effective than a single longer walk when it comes to lowering blood pressure. Taking those three walks after each meal could help reduce blood sugar spikes while simultaneously reducing blood pressure.

TIPS

IF YOU FEEL ANY DISCOMFORT, try waiting a few minutes.

There's no need to stride or march after a large meal: this is a promenade, not a power walk.

Pay attention to your posture, and remember to lift up from your hips. With a full stomach you don't want to be slumping.

Ambling in fading light after an evening meal? Follow the suggestions for night walking in Week 34: Walk Beneath a Full Moon (p. 39) and Week 46: Take a Night Walk (p. 190).

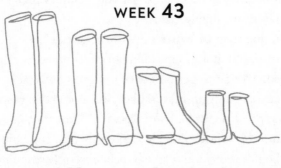

Walk with Others

FOR HUNDREDS OF YEARS THE Welsh hills rang with sound: clattering hooves, barking dogs, bellowing cattle, grunting pigs, honking geese. And, most distinctive of all, the peculiar high-pitched wail of drovers, the men (and occasionally women) who steered huge packs of livestock from Wales to London. The 200-mile journey may have been slow and laborious, but it was never lonely. Drovers walked in noisy packs that could be heard for miles around. Dozens of walkers accompanied them—boys taking up London apprenticeships, girls going into service, women visiting friends and family, cattle dealers, wealthy young men in search of adventure. These ramshackle throngs of people and animals wound through the landscape, eating together, sleeping together, moving together. Reading about drovers and their companions reminds us of the practical joys of *walking together*.

Anthropologists Tim Ingold and Jo Lee Vergunst describe walking as "a profoundly social activity." History confirms this: protests, parades, marches, processions, and pilgrimages have existed for centuries as convivial occasions, much like droving. Walking together provides safety and security. It stimulates conversation, fosters relationships, and cements friendships. Its slow, familiar pace makes it uniquely and incomparably inclusive.

Solo walking may be better suited to reflection (see Week 15: Walk Alone, p. 59), but group walking fulfills other fundamental human needs. Person-to-person contact triggers a cascade of feel-good chemicals, neurotransmitters like dopamine and oxytocin that protect us, as psychologist Susan Pinker says, "like a vaccine . . . now and well into the future." Merely shaking hands, she points out, floods our bodies and brains with oxytocin, instantly stripping away stress and anxiety. Over the last few years, and exacerbated by the COVID-19 pandemic, the case for being social has ballooned, proven not only by anecdotal evidence but by hundreds of academic studies: good social ties mean better physical, mental, and cognitive health, as well as a longer life.

The ill effects of loneliness are equally well documented. Numerous studies have linked it to depression and anxiety: a 2020 report suggests that lonely young people could be three times more likely to develop depression in the future, resulting in depressive symptoms that could last for years. Other studies have correlated loneliness with poor physical health. The lonely are more likely to suffer from dementia, heart disease, and stroke—with some experts claiming loneliness is as damaging as smoking, air pollution, and obesity.

But why walk in a group? Firstly, walking groups have been proven to develop the physical health of their members: reduced weight and body mass index (BMI) and lowered blood pressure and cholesterol (among other things) are routinely reported. More importantly, walking groups have impressively low dropout rates: when we walk together, we stay together.

But where walking groups excel is in the improved mental health of their members. A study involving 1,843 participants walking for a combined 74,000 hours found a "statistically significant" drop in feelings of stress and depression among regular group walkers, many of whom also reported greater feelings of satisfaction. So what is it about walking with others that makes us feel more satisfied?

Anthropologists Tessa Pollard and Stephanie Morris believe the shared experience of walking as a group can transform it from a pedestrian (excuse the pun) fitness session to a richly rewarding social occasion. Their studies suggest that when we walk with others, we experience feelings of social connection, acceptance, belonging, and safety. The slow rhythmic pace, the coordinated movement, and the absence of eye contact create a relaxed intimacy, making it easier to share and exchange confidences, thoughts, and ideas.

Meanwhile, the ebb and flow of walking in a group creates what anthropologists call *fleeting sociability*, now considered one of the primary factors making walking together so therapeutic. When we walk in company, we drift freely between individuals and conversations, shifting when we change direction or turn a corner, sometimes talking but sometimes walking in silent synchronicity. It's a very special mode of being in company and utterly unlike most social occasions. Pollard explains that it "makes for a transient and light form of social connection," that is particularly unintimidating.

There are other reasons that make walking together feel so uplifting. Pollard believes that the feeling of belonging engendered by group walking isn't only about being part of a crowd: "The feeling of belonging extends to the landscape itself." When we walk through a place—be it urban or rural—we connect with it in a very sensory way: we hear, smell, feel, even taste. Sharing this experience with others can make a group feel bonded both to one another and to the landscape. Moreover, we share our moments of accomplishment, of hunger, cold, curiosity, and wonder.

Pollard and Morris's own research involving women from deprived areas of Northern England found that walking groups were particularly effective for those facing turning points in their lives (social scientists call these biographical disruptions), when shared regular walks often became lifelines, spots of time that calmed, strengthened, and emboldened the walkers.

The twin traits of walking and talking have more in common than how the two words sound. In his book *The Body*, Bill Bryson speculates that *Homo sapiens* became bipedal around the same time as we developed communication skills. As little creatures hunting big creatures, he posits, our ability to communicate was almost as important as our ability to walk. Meanwhile, evolutionary biologist Daniel Lieberman notes that—thousands of years ago and in some tribes today—we foraged in groups and hunted in pairs. It's quite likely that our love of walking and talking in tandem is rooted deep in our DNA.

No surprise, then, that studies show the effects of group walking are enhanced when done in natural, rather than urban, environments. Researchers found that when walks took place in nature, they resulted in "a significant influence on mental well-being." Not a magic bullet, explained one study, "but a stepping stone to recovery."

In a study involving 1 percent of the adult female population of Australia, group hiking was frequently perceived as a source of psychological transformation and "emotional rescue," in which the togetherness was as crucial a factor as the wild landscape. Group walking in the Australian bush guaranteed safety while providing camaraderie, often resulting in friendships that lasted for years afterward. Many of this study's participants reported remarkable "flow-on" effects: hikers returned believing they were, as one respondent put it, "a nicer person, mother and wife."

TIPS

NEUROSCIENTIST DANIEL LEVITIN SAYS HIKING, new places, and fresh faces keep our brains youthful, and a group walking vacation combines all three.

Your physician can direct you to dedicated walking groups for specific health conditions, as can support groups. Or check out Walk with a Doc (walkwithadoc.org).

Local libraries are a good source of information, while numerous organizations run group hikes/treks. Try Meetup (meetup.com).

Charities often organize fundraising walks.

Consider making a pilgrimage—often the epitome of social walking (see Week 40: Walk Like a Pilgrim, p. 165).

Unsure whether to walk with others or alone? Science journalist Florence Williams suggests "if you are depressed or anxious, social walking in nature boosts your mood . . . if you want to solve problems in your life, self-reflect and jot your creativity, it's better to go alone."

WEEK **44**

Seek Out the Sublime

ONE HOT SUMMER AFTERNOON IN 2014, I was walking in the rock caves of Bohemia when a storm whipped up from nowhere. The air darkened and grew thick with electricity. Bolts of silver lightning zipped through the sky. And in the eerie charged light, the huge pale rocks glimmered and trembled, their mossy seams a luminous elfin green. It was a mesmerizing moment during which my mind emptied of all thought. And yet I felt not empty but gripped by a feeling I couldn't articulate. Later, I learned that the emotion holding me spellbound during that strangely intoxicating time had a name: awe.

We've all had moments like this. Moments of intense wonder at the astonishing mystery and intoxicating beauty of a landscape or place. The first glimpse of a mountain range, a glorious blaze of sunset, the sudden sighting of a waterfall—each of us carries these memories within us, often recalling them with unusual clarity. We may feel deeply moved, even altered, by these experiences. For some, these moments have a spiritual or religious significance. Frequently—although not always—these moments occur when we're out in nature.

Frequently—although not always—our response is tinged with fear or incredulity.

This isn't a new phenomenon: poets and philosophers have been documenting the power of the sublime for hundreds of years. But recently, awe has become the subject of scientific study. In several universities, neuroscientists and psychologists are diligently exploring the effects of awe both from their laboratories and from the wilderness—with fascinating results.

But what do we mean by awe? The psychologist Michelle Shiota describes it as a state of mindfulness effortlessly ignited (unlike meditation) and thrillingly unexpected, an experience that makes us feel humbler and smaller, but with the power to change us in some way. Shiota noticed, in early experiments, that awe wasn't signaled by smiling but by mild expressions of shock—widened eyes, raised eyebrows, dropped jaws. She also noticed that awe-inducing scenes changed the brains of observers. During a series of experiments in which participants were subjected to a range of scenes and were then asked to critique a piece of written work, Shiota found that those who felt awe subsequently demonstrated stronger analytical skills and more rigorous thought processes. Other researchers reported the same outcome: being exposed to awe was linked to better cognitive processing. Professor Melanie Rudd argued that awe expands our sense of time, enabling us to better focus our attention. Rudd wondered if this sharper focus accounted for the correlation between awe and better cognition. When she exposed individuals to awe, she noted that they felt less time-pressured, less impatient, than their non-awed counterparts.

Meanwhile, another researcher in psychology, Dacher Keltner, wondered how else awe might change us. His experiments showed that exposure to awe-inducing scenes engendered greater feelings of humility, curiosity, happiness, and altruism. In one of his experiments, people who had gazed at awe-provoking trees were more likely to pick up purposely dropped pens than were participants who gazed at a building. Later experiments found that awe facilitated feelings of belonging, making participants feel more emotionally connected to one another and better able to deal with uncertainty.

The most intriguing experiments were those conducted by Dr. Jennifer Stellar. Stellar exposed participants to a range of scenes, then took saliva samples, testing for a pro-inflammatory cytokine called interleukin-6 (IL-6), a signaling molecule associated with many chronic inflammatory diseases and with depression. Bizarrely, Stellar found that participants who had experienced the greatest feelings of awe also had the lowest levels of IL-6. Wonder, more than any other positive emotion, appeared to improve physical well-being. "Awe," she wrote in her report, "was the strongest predictor of lower levels of pro-inflammatory cytokines."

No surprise then that the United States has pioneered awe walks—short, partially guided strolls where a walker's attention is directed to significant trees, cloud formations, or lakes, or in cities, to spectacular buildings or sight lines. Studies of guided awe walkers found them feeling more positive after eight weeks than walkers who hadn't been awe-guided. Better still, the effect was cumulative, suggesting that the more we seek out awe while walking, the greater our potential well-being.

No one needs a guided awe walk. All we have to do is turn off our phones, use our senses, and take note of the bewitching beauty that turns up on almost every walk, often in the smallest of things—lichen, moss, insects, raindrops. Anyone can cultivate the capacity to marvel.

TIPS

WHEN YOUR THOUGHTS FLOAT BACK to your to-do list, nudge them away, scan the horizon, smell the air, listen.

Studies indicate that novelty is an important component of awe, so try walking somewhere new, walking backward (see Week 49, p. 202), at night (Weeks 34, p. 139, and 46, p. 190), or barefoot (Week 29, p. 119).

Experiencing something new on our regular walks isn't as difficult as it sounds—few of us look up at the sky, but cloud formations are often staggeringly handsome.

Binoculars or a magnifying glass make it easier to spot smaller wondrous details.

Seek out the work of naturalists and nature writers, who can alert us to the miraculous spots of sublimity we might not otherwise notice. Knowledge doesn't counter mystery: it enlarges it.

A 2019 study found that people rated as curious (by themselves and their friends) were more likely to experience the sublime. Nurture your curiosity with Week 21: Exercise Your Curiosity Muscle—Walk a Ley Line (p. 84).

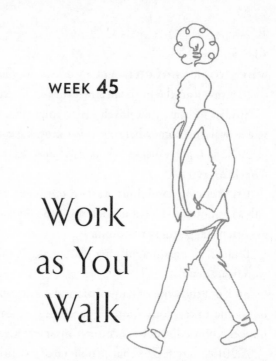

Work as You Walk

FIVE YEARS AGO I WAS on the brink of giving up my job as a (very sedentary) writer and researcher. My lower back pain made long periods of sitting impossible—and if I couldn't sit, how could I work? Costly treatment from physiotherapists and osteopaths had failed. An expensive orthopedic chair had failed. A program of back-strengthening exercises had failed. The only time I was pain-free was when I walked. I was just about to switch careers and become a walking-tour guide when I opened a magazine and saw a photograph of Victoria Beckham on a treadmill. But this was not any old treadmill. Ms. Beckham—elegantly attired in spiked heels and a chic long jacket, not a flash of Lycra in sight—was on a tread-mill desk.

My interest was piqued, but I had my doubts. Wouldn't I fall off? Weren't they stupidly expensive? And where would I put a moving desk the size of a sofa? The question that really gnawed at me was more complicated: How would walking with a laptop affect my body, my brain, and my writing? A year later, still racked with back pain, I bought a treadmill desk.

Walking as you work inevitably burns more calories than sitting. A fairly standard speed of 1.5 mph on a treadmill desk typically burns five times more calories than sitting at a desk. At a walking desk, we will—on average—add an additional 2,000 steps to our daily step count.

Walking as you work (sometimes called deskercising) has a proven physiological impact, quite simply because it enables us to swap sedentary time for active time. Studies show that deskercisers achieve weight loss and fat loss, reduced hip and waist circumference, lowered total cholesterol, reduced blood glucose and insulin levels, and lowered blood pressure.

But the results go beyond the physiological. Researchers have found that using a treadmill desk improves our short-term memory and attention. In a 2015 study, two groups of people were asked to read a lengthy document and a series of emails. One group worked at treadmill desks (set at 1.4 mph), while the other group sat at traditional desks. Electrodes were attached to their scalps monitoring the electrical activity of their brains as they read, a process known as EEG testing. After forty minutes both groups were questioned on the contents of the documents and emails. The treadmill workers had better recall, remembering more of what they had read than their nonwalking counterparts.

But the treadmill workers also experienced greater self-perceived on-task attention, meaning they felt more focused, more attentive to the task in hand. So were they actually working with increased concentration? The EEG results suggested they were, revealing additional activity in the brain parts associated with memory and attention. Other reports have since confirmed that working while walking improves our visual working memory (the bit responsible for absorbing information and using it to make decisions) while reducing the number of errors we make.

This isn't all . . . An earlier study from the University of Minnesota tracked forty office workers who, after a year of treadmill-desking, became both more productive and more creative. Dr. Avner Ben-Ner, the lead researcher, attributed this to the increased blood flow to the brain, adding, "If you are slumped in your chair, you don't get as much benefit from your brain."

Ben-Ner's findings reflect an experiment from Stanford University in which office workers were tested on their ability to think divergently—first while seated at tables and then while pacing on a treadmill desk. Eighty-one percent of the participants were more creative, sparking many more ideas while walking than while seated.

The link between physical activity and divergent original thinking is now well established, with numerous studies concluding that movement stimulates creativity, provoking new ideas in greater quantity and of greater quality. In his book *In Praise of Walking*, Shane O'Mara argues that "we can reach a more creative state while being in motion," speculating that not only does walking put our brain into better physiological condition but that it opens up the entire brain network, including "far-flung" corners. As networks and pathways open, we can "zoom in and out" of thoughts, memories, sensations—drawing on multiple experiences and making novel connections that facilitate lateral thought.

Studies now suggest that how we move can enhance our creativity still further. A 2020 Japanese experiment in which sixty-three female students were asked to come up with ideas for using a newspaper, either while moving their arms with loose, fluid movements or while moving their arms with angular movements, found those with smooth, flowing arms came up with significantly more ideas. The study authors concluded that "fluidity enacted by arm movements robustly enhances creative fluency." My takeaway from this?

Swing your arms (as described in Week 2: Improve Your Gait, p. 10) and don't hold back!

I can't honestly say that I'm any more creative or divergent while working on a treadmill desk. But of one thing I am certain: the back pain that plagued my life has gone. Instead of becoming a tour guide, I'm still researching and writing books—much of which I do at my walking desk.

TIPS

DESKERCISING TAKES A BIT OF getting used to and may not be for everyone. Either way, press your employer to invest in a few treadmill desks.

Try before you buy, making sure the desk is fully adjustable and that the desk space is sufficiently sized for your needs. Treadmill desks are large and extremely heavy, so choose its location with care, avoiding sunny windows and overly warm spaces.

Start slow. Most deskercisers walk at a speed between 0.3 and 1.5 mph.

Once you're used to your treadmill desk, change the speed according to the nature of your work. I increase the pace when I'm reading (2 mph) and slow it when I'm typing (1.5 mph) and thinking (1 mph).

Intersperse time at your treadmill desk with time sitting at a normal desk. And pay attention to which desk—walking or sitting—works best, according to the work you're doing.

No treadmill desk? Organize *walking* meetings and *strolling* brainstorms. Pace the corridors, pavements, and parking lots whenever possible. Even very short walks have been shown to "open up the free flow of ideas" according to Marily Oppezzo, whose pioneering experiments also found that, for the very best results, a walk should be taken outside.

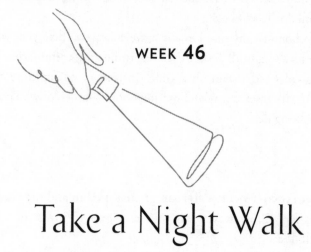

Take a Night Walk

IN 1994, AN EARTHQUAKE CUT the power lines in the city of Los Angeles, plunging the city into darkness. Panicked residents began calling the local emergency centers. Not because their houses were toppling over, but because there were strange alien happenings in the night sky that many callers described as "a giant silvery cloud." The anxious inhabitants of L.A. were seeing—for the very first time—the Milky Way.

At the same time but on the other side of the world, an Australian mum was growing increasingly frustrated. Keen to exercise but with no free daylight time, Di Westaway made the bold decision to night hike with a few girlfriends. With head lamps in place, Westaway and her friends began meeting once a week to walk deep into the Australian bush. Initially their three-hour hikes were focused on exercising. But Westaway quickly realized that their night forays were reconnecting them to wilderness, silence, and most important, the dense velvet darkness of the bush at night. "We thought it was exercise we needed but, looking back, the night sky and the darkness were equally important," she recalled.

Nighttime sky glow is now brighter than ever, exacerbated by low-cost LED lights, which have flooded our dark skies with far-reaching blue light. Today more than 99 percent of Americans and Europeans live under skies so light-polluted that the Milky Way is virtually invisible. Some of us live beneath a haze so permanently bright our eyes *never* switch to night-vision mode.

And yet darkness is a fundamental human need. Research suggests its deficit could be linked to depression, insomnia, obesity, weakened immunity, and heart disease. Laboratory experiments have revealed how exposure to light at night disrupts circadian and neuroendocrine physiology, potentially speeding up tumor growth. When Israeli scientists placed satellite photos showing artificial night light over a map of breast-cancer cases, the results were shocking: the lighter the location at night, the greater the prevalence of breast cancer. In neighborhoods where it was bright enough to read a book at night, women had a 73 percent higher risk of developing breast cancer.

Nor is it only bright light that appears to be affecting us. According to Dr. Eva Selhub, "even low levels of night light can reduce brain plasticity and interfere with normal brain cell structures." Researchers now think that night light inhibits our production of melatonin, the hormone that helps us sleep. Sleep researcher Christina Pierpaoli Parker told *National Geographic* magazine that night walking helps us sleep, "by acting on the homeostatic sleep drive." Either way, it's clear that we need darkness "to survive and thrive," as a leading American medical council put it.

Nocturnal ambles and night hikes reacquaint us with starlight, moonbeams, and darkness, introducing us to landscapes that feel familiar but are at once entirely new, and simultaneously recalibrating our body clocks according to the light/dark cycles we've lived with for millennia.

Governments, helped by organizations like the International Dark-Sky Association, have started identifying and designating areas of darkness—pristine night skies where we can see thousands of stars. To experience the full benefits of darkness, go to darksky.org and find the dark skies nearest to you. We don't need to travel far to experience a night walk in all its splendor, but the less light pollution, the more authentic our night walk, and the greater our chances of seeing shooting stars, meteors, or comets. It's not only the night sky that comes alive in the dark. According to sea-life expert Heather Buttivant, night is the very best time to see rock pools in action. Take a UV flashlight and watch seaweed and anemones glow and glimmer in neon hues of red, blue, green, pink, and purple.

Night walking comes with its own risks, which can be minimized by choosing a route that's easily navigable, flat, and even beneath the foot. You don't want to be scrambling over rocks (unless you're rock-pooling, of course) or tripping in rabbit holes. Avoid wet nights, as you don't want to be slipping and sliding. For stargazing you need an uninterrupted sight line, making open lands preferable to forests.

Your first night walk is best taken in territory you know well. Rest assured it will look splendidly different at night! Set out while it's still light to give your eyes time to adjust: dusk is ideal. If you take the same route there and back you can make a mental note of dimmed landmarks, meaning less chance of getting lost on your return, when it might be pitch-black.

TIPS

TAKE A HEAD LAMP WITH a red-light setting to protect your vision. If the head lamp has a dimmer switch or a range of brightness settings, all the better. A head lamp leaves your hands free to fumble with a map or a hip flask and can double as a hanging lamp for your night picnic. But a head lamp won't help your eyes adjust to night vision, so don't use it if you don't need to.

The temperature invariably falls at night, so dress in layers. Wear boots or shoes with good grip—you want to be spotting comets and night creatures, not worrying about your feet. Avoid flapping clothing or anything you might trip over.

It's easier to stumble at night: take trekking poles or a stick.

Take a fully charged phone for emergencies and, unless you're very brave or foolhardy, a friend or two. If you want to see wildlife, limit the size of group and use your eyes rather than a head lamp.

If darkness has already fallen, sit inside in the dark for at least twenty minutes to allow your eyes to adjust without straining. Avoid looking at very bright light (car headlights, for example), which make it much harder for our eyes to adjust to the darkness. Pressure applied to the eyes speeds up the process of switching to night vision, so try pressing your hands gently against your sockets.

Night vision is demanding—and the older we are, the more demanding it is—so rest your eyes regularly by cupping them with your palms. Seeing in the dark is all about peripheral vision, which means focusing on the sides and edges of things rather than their centers.

If you're planning a night walk in an official Dark Sky–accredited site (and who wouldn't?), take advice on your route or walk it first in daylight.

Sound travels much farther at night. Listen for the sounds you won't hear during daylight hours—owls hooting, cars on distant roads, the scurrying of nocturnal creatures.

Take a flask of something hot, or a hip flask, if it's cold.

Want to stargaze? Invest in a pair of astronomy binoculars, and download a stargazing mobile app for identifying celestial bodies.

Rather go with an organized group? Search online for guided night hikes, bat hikes, or nightingale walks (sometimes organized by wildlife charities). Astronomy societies often hold stargazing walks, and a few cities hold Reclaim the Night walks (sometimes women only).

Wherever you are, slow down: a night walk is not a step-counting power walk but a chance to wander and wonder.

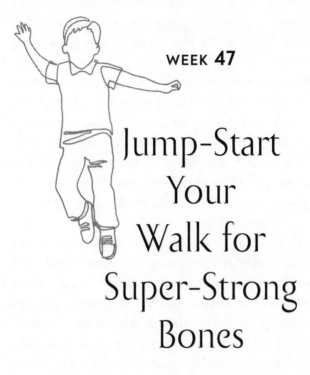

Jump-Start Your Walk for Super-Strong Bones

EVERY YEAR, IN THE REMOTE desert plains of Yemen, not far from the Red Sea, a sporting competition takes place. This astonishing and barely believable event is a rite of passage for the young men of the Zaraniq tribe. Without gyms, sports coaches, or cushioned footwear, the men leap—effortlessly and gracefully—over a row of 6- to 7-foot camels in a single bound. The Zaraniq don't use weapons to battle their enemies. Instead, they rely on their stamina and strength, manifested in camel-jumping competitions.

According to evolutionary biologist Daniel Lieberman, our bodies were built to leap, jump, and bound. Hence we have springy arches in our feet and an Achilles tendon, which helps propel us into the air. Running, dancing, and speed walking are all forms of locomotion in which we spring from one foot to the other, carrying our own body weight as we move and working against gravity. Unlike swimming or cycling, all three are excellent weight-bearing exercise.

Regular walking is very effective for *preserving* our bones. Like our muscles, our bones begin weakening as we approach our thirties. Unsurprisingly, our sedentary lifestyles mean that osteoporosis (which translates as porous bone) and its precursor, osteopenia (early bone thinning), now affect 55 percent of Americans over the age of fifty—male and female. When osteoporosis sets in, we can no longer rely on our bones to carry us: even the smallest of bends or jolts can snap or fracture a piece of our skeleton.

But can regular walking *build* (rather than merely preserve) our bone mineral density (BMD)? Yes—but only if we modify our usual stroll. Bone is a living tissue, able to rebuild itself throughout our lives—a process known as remodeling. For our bones to remodel themselves as stronger and denser, they need the shock of ground impact. The greater the impact, the better our bones. Velocity also plays a part: the faster we move, the greater the impact as our foot hits the ground, multiplying the bone benefits still further.

For this reason, running often beats walking when it comes to building new bone. Brisk walking is better than strolling: a study involving more than 60,000 postmenopausal women found that those who walked briskly at least four times a week had a lower risk of hip fractures than women who either didn't walk or walked less often or more slowly.

Even better, add some bounding to your walk. The very best exercise we can do to both build and preserve our bones is to jump. Researchers at Brigham Young University found that a few minutes of jumping was more effective at building strong bones than anything else, including running. Moreover, they found that jumping ten times a day significantly improved bone mineral density after a mere two months. Other studies reflect this: jumping strengthens the bones of teenagers, men, cyclists, rats—just about everyone. Skipping (without a rope) has similar effects and makes a wonderful interlude when walking.

There's another very important reason for introducing other movements into your walking routine. When we *mix up* movement— adding in sudden changes of direction—our bones respond favorably, becoming even stronger. Athletes who play soccer or racket sports have better bone density than those who don't—and that includes long-distance runners. Indeed, studies show the bone strength of movers who mix it up to be on a par with high jumpers. Researchers believe this is due to frequent switching of direction: racket and soccer players move not only forward but backward and sideways, as well as stopping and starting. Scientists refer to mixed-up movement using the catchy (ahem) phrase *odd-impact exercise loading*. Adding in additional movement—like dancing, skipping, backward walking, or jumping—transforms our daily walk into a powerful feat of bone building.

Countryside walks offer numerous chances for bounding or leaping. Rocks, fallen branches, streams, and ditches are ideal excuses to leap. We can bound over puddles and jump from stiles.

On city walks, we can (respectfully) leap over gravestones in cemeteries, spring across flower beds in parks, vault low walls, and bound up steps.

If you don't fancy interspersing your walk with jumping, skipping, or hopping (not recommended for the frail or elderly), keep a brisk pace. A recent study found that walking at 3 to 4 mph was the perfect pace for preserving bone density in the elderly. For bone building, add a few sharp changes of direction, some sidestepping and backward walking (see Week 49: Walk Backward, p. 202), maintaining the same energetic pace.

Nordic walking, hill walking, rucking, and weighted walking (Weeks 43, 38, and 36 pp. 177, 157, and 148) can also convert a daily saunter into a bone-building workout, particularly when done in sunshine. Intriguing new research suggests that heat may protect against bone loss, perhaps explaining why the incidence of hip fractures is greater in northern countries than in southern countries.

TIPS

TRY STARTING AND ENDING YOUR walk with ten jumps, done in the privacy of your own home.

Find jumping tiring? Drink a cup of coffee an hour before you plan to start. A 2021 study showed that caffeine aided and enhanced jumping. (Indeed, most forms of movement are eased and accelerated with a shot of caffeine.)

Can't maintain a brisk walking speed? Try increasing your speed for a minute, or between trees or lampposts, then slow down again.

Walk with children who will—without the least self-consciousness—welcome the chance to skip and jump. This has the added bonus of building their bones, helping them prevent bone loss in their old age. It may not be in your lifetime, but one day they will thank you.

WEEK **48**

Walk Hungry

IT MAY SEEM COUNTERINTUITIVE TO suggest walking when we're at our most hungry. Surely we need food to fuel all those steps? But no, quite the reverse. The latest science suggests that a well-paced walk *before* breakfast—while our body is still in fasting mode—burns more fat, improves the way in which our body responds to insulin, and cuts our risk of type 2 diabetes and heart disease. The time to eat breakfast, it appears, is *after* we've walked. There's one exception: long, demanding hikes. In which case you should stoke up with a good breakfast.

Sports scientists now think that exercise regulates our appetite, so the more we move, the less we crave superfluous food. A 2019 study found that healthy young men who exercised before breakfast consumed less food during the day than on days when they ate breakfast and did no exercise (or on the days when they exercised *after* breakfast). Another study found that overweight men who walked for sixty minutes *before* breakfast burned double the amount of fat as those exercising *after* breakfast. Six weeks later an even more dramatic change became apparent: the before-breakfast exercisers had better control of their blood sugar and insulin levels. According to the researchers, the muscles of those exercising on an empty stomach displayed a greater number of the proteins needed to shift glucose out of their blood and into their muscles. Which is to say, their bodies were healthier and worked more efficiently. Indeed, the researchers described the changes incurred by exercising pre-breakfast as "positive and profound."

A 2020 study found that low-intensity exercise—like walking—is particularly effective when done while fasting, with low-intensity exercisers burning more weight than vigorous (or high-intensity) exercisers. The authors suggested that low-intensity movement before breakfast may even help curb inflammation, which is responsible for so much contemporary disease, from Alzheimer's to cancer. Why might this happen? Researchers aren't sure, but it's possibly because fat secretes inflammatory modules that fuel chronic inflammation, making fasted walking not just for those looking to shed weight. The record-breaking athlete and coach Colin Jackson starts every morning with a fasted walk, covering 3.7 miles in fifty minutes.

I too do a fasted walk every morning, and it's become an essential part of my day. It's very simple: get up, have a glass of water, put on your athletic shoes, and walk. Bingo!

If you want to lose weight, follow Jackson's example and do a fasted walk every morning at the same time. Research published in *Obesity* in 2019 suggests that the key to weight loss lies in habit and consistency: those walking at the same time every day were more successful in keeping weight off.

TIPS

WALKING ON AN EMPTY STOMACH can take adjusting to, particularly if you're used to an early breakfast. Start with short walks and build up slowly.

Can't walk while hungry? Try eating a banana or some nuts and dried fruit beforehand.

While studies suggest that fasted walking is particularly effective for reducing obesity, it's not for everyone. Listen to your body or consult your physician.

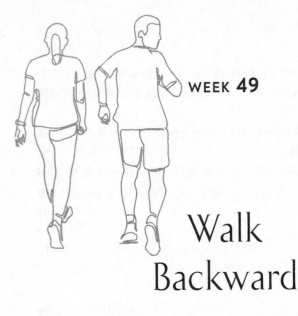

WEEK **49**

Walk
Backward

ON MARCH 7, 1931, A Texan called Plennie Wingo arrived, backward, at a rodeo in Fort Worth. Dressed in a cowboy outfit, a tangle of advertising signs around his neck, Wingo announced his plan to walk the world—in reverse. He'd been practicing for six months, walking backward for twenty minutes every night, under cover of darkness so that no one would steal his idea. A month later he set off, wearing glasses with miniature mirrors attached to the side of each lens so that he could see where he was going. A stout stick helped him balance. Wingo's little-known story is both ludicrous and hair-raising. From Texas he walked, backward, into Oklahoma, then Missouri, then Illinois, covering fifteen to twenty miles a day. In two months he had worn through sixteen pairs of metal toeplates.

His reverse walk continued: Ohio, Connecticut, then Boston, where he caught a ship to Hamburg, arriving in January alongside squalls of snow. Through ice and snow, he walked to Berlin, Dresden, Prague, and into Romania, Bulgaria, and Turkey, where he was promptly and pitilessly thrown into jail. He eventually finished his journey, having clocked up 7,000 miles, assuring him a place in *The Guinness Book of World Records*. By all accounts Wingo should have died on his madcap journey. Instead, he lived to the age of ninety-eight, regularly walking backward and always maintaining that it was "good for health."

Was Wingo right? It appears that he was. In the last few decades, backward walking has emerged as a breathtakingly simple, little-known means of improving our fitness. In fact, studies show that the best way to improve our forward walking is—perversely—by walking backward. According to a 2020 study published in *Brain Communications*, this is because when we walk in reverse, we use a completely different team of core and lower body muscles. Strengthening these helps our entire lower body to work effectively and efficiently.

But backward walking also enhances our forward walking by improving our balance and stability. When we walk without using our eyes to guide us, we need a sophisticated grasp of the space we're moving through and stepping into—something called proprioception, kinesthesia, or even our "sixth sense." This relies on our proprioceptors, neurons embedded in our joints, muscles, and limbs, which work alongside our senses to communicate with our central nervous system and our brain—an almost miraculous chain of instructions that takes place in a nanosecond, fine-tuned over millions of years so we can walk with minimal mental exertion. This intricately coordinated chain of neuromuscular commands happens hundreds of times every day—when our feet dodge a sudden hole or change tread to accommodate concrete pavement, gravel or bog (for instance), or when we leap for a ball or dash down a darkened flight of steps. Researchers speculate that because backward walking demands such complex unfamiliar movement patterns, it enhances our proprioceptive abilities, thereby improving our balance, as well as sharpening our senses.

Researchers have also established that backward walking is more physically demanding, exercising our lower body muscles more thoroughly than when we move forward. Walking in reverse, we land on our toes before rolling through to our heel—which is why Wingo constantly wore out the steel toecaps on his shoes. By landing on our toes, we engage our shin muscles and our glutes, as well as our rectus femoris (one of our quadriceps muscles), making them work infinitely harder than they work when our legs move forward. All things considered, backward walking provides an excellent aerobic workout, crunching through more calories than forward walking.

Early research suggests that backward walking also makes our hamstrings more flexible as well as benefits our posture. Normally, when we walk, we lean forward slightly. But reverse walking prevents this, nudging our spine and core to work harder in order that we keep upright and stable—and realigning our pelvis in the process. Which may explain why a 2011 study found that ten minutes of reverse walking, four times a week, reduced lower back pain after only three weeks.

Other studies have linked backward walking to improved speed, stride, and gait. When we walk in reverse, we strengthen our knee joints and our quadriceps—both of which help our gait (meaning that we are better coordinated, more fluid and elegant in our movements, and able to walk with more ease and less effort). For this reason, backward walking has had excellent results for people with impaired movement, including those with juvenile rheumatoid arthritis, knee osteoarthritis, strokes, Parkinson's disease, cerebral palsy, multiple sclerosis, and spinal or knee injuries.

Increased confidence, strength, agility, sleep, and mood have also been reported after training in backward walking, as has better mental focus. A study of children with ADHD found that after walking backward for ten minutes, they could concentrate for longer, producing fewer mistakes in their subsequent work. Whether this works more universally remains to be seen, but it's possible that the greater ability to focus is a spillover result of the intense concentration required while walking in reverse. As the researchers wrote, backward walking could "improve attentive performance."

I was determined to try backward walking for myself, having examined such compelling evidence. And what a joy it was! When we move in reverse—walking out of a landscape—the vista widens rather than narrows. With every step we take, the space around us expands and unfolds, revealing itself slowly and mysteriously. It's quite unlike walking into a landscape, where the scene ahead of us can appear unchanged for hours.

Without eyes to guide us, our other senses spring into action. We become vividly aware of our body moving through space. With our attention fully focused on the place and press of each step, we feel the ground beneath our toes, the backward roll of each foot, the direction of the wind. In our all-encompassing attempt to stay safe and upright, our mind cannot stray or wander (no drifting reflections, dramatic epiphanies, or scintillating conversation). When we walk forward, we can forget our body and exist solely in our mind. But when we walk backward, we abandon the mind and exist solely in our body.

TIPS

WINGO SPRAINED AND FRACTURED HIS ankle on at least two occasions, as well as caused a car crash. Be careful: find an even, familiar, unoccupied stretch on which to practice, and start slowly. Alternatively, ask someone to guide you.

Focus on each step (start small), landing on your toes and rolling back to your heel. Try to include a few minutes of backward walking in your daily walk

Turn to Week 20: Walk to Remember (p. 80) to see how backward walking can also improve your memory.

Minimalist footwear (see Week 29: Walk Barefoot, p. 119) gives us a better physical sense of the terrain, which enhances the full sensory experience of walking backward.

Studying a subject requiring the full force of your brain? Fascinating investigations from the Huberman Lab found that a few minutes spent in unaccustomed unstable movement—like backward walking—prompted the brain to release neurochemicals accelerating plasticity and making it significantly easier to learn and remember. Note: This works only while the movement is novel. It won't work for regular reverse walkers.

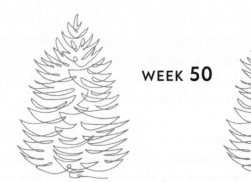

Walk in an Evergreen Forest (for a Good Night's Sleep)

IN 1795, MARY WOLLSTONECRAFT ARRIVED in Norway. Penniless and unhappy, and carrying her illegitimate baby, Wollstonecraft spent time walking through Norway's famous pine forests. In a letter to her lover, she wrote: "I am more alive than you have seen me in a long, long time." Her letters spoke elatedly of the "wild perfume" of the "pines and firs" that had "soothed her heart." Wollstonecraft, arguably the inventor of feminism with her ground-breaking book, *A Vindication of the Rights of Women*, believed her Norwegian trip had helped "turn a new page in the history of my own heart."

Wollstonecraft may have been one of the first to write about the spectacular power of the pine tree, but Native Americans, the Chinese, and the Koreans have been using the pine tree as a source of medicine for centuries, while the Greeks and Romans believed pine nuts to be a sort of latter-day Viagra. So it should come as no surprise that today's researchers are catching up, using saliva tests, blood tests, and neuroimaging techniques to prove the miraculous therapeutic effects of the pine tree—which includes any conifer in the genus *Pinus* of the Pinaceae family (cedars, spruces, firs, larches, hemlocks, and pines).

The pine tree's secret weapon is its arsenal of essential oils called phytoncides, chemical compounds created by the tree to defend itself from attacks by insects, animals, fungi, and disease. When we walk into a pine forest and smell that distinctive resinous aroma, we're smelling the trees' self-defense systems—their phytoncides spraying into the air, rather like hundreds of aerosols being pumped simultaneously.

Every tree—indeed, every plant—produces its own unique cocktail of self-defending compounds, some of which have proven to be anti-inflammatory, antibacterial, antifungal, and antioxidant (see Week 19: Amble amid Trees, p. 75). Pine trees produce certain phytoncides in abundance, and forest expert Peter Wohlleben claims the air in a pine forest is the cleanest air we will ever breathe.

For me, the most intriguing experiments involving pine trees are not to do with cleanliness, but with sleep. The first researchers to spot a connection between pine trees and improved sleep were a team of Japanese scientists who, in 2005, discovered that a phytoncide called alpha-pinene (α-pinene) caused rats to sleep for longer than normal. Subsequent experiments found that alpha-pinene acted exactly as a sleeping pill does, following the same chemical pathways but without any side effects and without affecting the delta activity necessary for deep sleep. Commonly used sleep medication increases sleep quantity but at the expense of quality, because it reduces delta activity. (Delta waves occur during deep sleep.) Rodents inhaling or consuming alpha-pinene slept more deeply and for longer.

The phytoncides of conifers are made up of chemicals called terpenes. While alpha-pinene is the most abundant, the second most abundant, 3-Carene, has also been linked to improved sleep in rodents. In other words, pine trees produce at least two sleep-inducing compounds.

Experiments have now started on humans, with promising results. In a 2019 Korean study, a group of cancer patients spent six days in a forest predominantly of cedar, cypress, and larch trees, enjoying what the Japanese call *shinrin-yoku* (forest bathing), including a daily thirty-minute walk. At the end of the trial their sleep efficiency (the amount of time in bed spent sleeping rather than tossing and turning) had improved. They were also sleeping for longer.

A second study found that the sleep-inducing benefits of walking in a pine forest were enhanced if the walk was taken in the afternoon. In this Japanese study, the walks taken were two hours long, and participants were asked to take some before midday and some in the afternoon. Both groups improved their shut-eye, but the longest sleeps were reserved for the afternoon walkers.

Like Mary Wollstonecraft, I have been lucky enough to wander through a Norwegian forest of conifers, breathing in the thickly perfumed air and experiencing similar feelings of rejuvenation. In the summer months I hiked and collected bilberries (traditional summer activities in Scandinavia), returning in the winter to snow walk. In the suppressing cold of a Nordic winter, the conifer smell was more elusive. According to *shinrin-yoku* pioneer and researcher Dr. Qing Li, forest bathing can be done at any time, although the concentration of phytoncides will be at its highest when the temperature hits 86°F.

But new research indicates that this may not always be the case. Terpene emissions are affected by various factors in addition to temperature: amount and duration of daylight, season, and the trees' age. A Korean study found that some forests emitted more terpenes in September, while those in other locations released more in May.

Some forests emitted more at night, while others secreted more during the day. According to this study, the only consistencies lay with old trees and wind: older trees produce fewer terpenes, and wind always disperses terpenes.

Terpenes do more than help us sleep. A Danish 2021 meta-analysis found evidence of reduced inflammation and improved immunity after "breathing in nature-derived compounds." Thirty minutes a week was sufficient to cut levels of blood pressure and depression . . . although optimal results peaked at four hours.

TIPS

TO IMPROVE YOUR SLEEP, WALK in the afternoon—and inhale deeply, through the nose. Or try the perfumer's technique of taking a series of short, sharp inhalations.

Seek out natural evergreen forests rather than commercial pine forests. The greater the variety of conifers, the greater the diversity of phytoncides.

For optimal terpene count, walk on a warm, windless day and make a beeline for forests containing younger trees.

Other woodlands have benefits (see Week 19: Amble amid Trees, p. 75), so don't worry if there's nothing evergreen on your doorstep.

No trees near you? Don't be defeated: a study from Northwestern University found that insomniac women who walked regularly on a treadmill extended their nightly sleep by forty-five minutes.

Countries with extensive pine forests include Scotland, Germany, Canada, parts of the United States (especially Alaska), Tasmania, Korea, Poland, and—of course—Japan. Consider a hiking break (see Week 36: Walk with a Pack, p. 148) or an eco-therapy break. Some forests now offer guided forest bathing sessions.

Many writers have extolled the smell of pine forest, but my favorite description is Nan Shepherd's: "like strawberry jam on the boil."

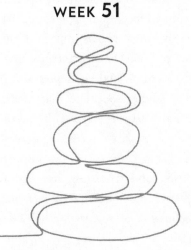

Walking as Meditation

ONCE, WHEN I WAS WALKING in New Mexico, lost and map-less, I accidentally stumbled into a Zen Buddhist center and found myself in the midst of a walking meditation. As the monks circumambulated—slowly, silently, barefoot in their black robes—I watched in astonishment. For years I had flirted with meditation, relishing the idea of existing utterly in the present. But sitting with my eyes closed made me sleepy, and when my spine instructed me to sit less and walk more, I gave up meditation altogether. Watching this supremely graceful walking meditation, in which the monks used the rhythm of their steps to reach an (apparent) inner stillness, compelled me to revisit mediation—on foot.

Dozens of studies indicate that meditation can counter the stresses of everyday life—stresses that, left unchecked, often leave deep and lasting marks, from raised blood pressure and inflammation to poor immunity, insomnia, depression, and anxiety. A review of sixteen studies investigating the impact of meditation on nurses (a group typically "plagued by stress and burnout") found that meditation helped with stress, anxiety, depression, burnout, empathy, and mood. Other studies speculate that meditation (seated and moving) can prevent and even reverse the detrimental effects of a stressful environment, in part—according to biologist Sabrina Venditti at Rome's Sapienza University—by "improving [our] immune system, metabolism, and stress-response pathways." Meditation, says Venditti, who uses the eloquent term *molecules of silence*, appears to alter us at a cellular level, turning on helpful genes and turning off harmful genes.

But meditation isn't only for those suffering from stress, burnout, or ill health. It's also been found to structurally change parts of the brain, strengthening the prefrontal cortex (the brain region involved in planning and decision-making), enlarging the hippocampus (our memory store), and shrinking the amygdala (the part of our brains linked to fear and anxiety). Brain scans show that regular meditators have denser gray matter (the tissue containing brain cells), a predictor of intelligence.

Sara Lazar, a neuroscientist at Harvard University, runs a lab devoted to studying the effects of meditation on the brain. After an experiment involving meditators and copious amounts of brain scanning, Lazar discovered answers to the questions on everybody's lips: How long must we meditate to alter the structure of our brains—years or months? And how often should we be meditating—weekly, daily, or hourly? And for how long—hours or minutes?

Lazar's findings took her by surprise: in only eight weeks, participants with no previous experience of meditating had expanded critical areas of their brain. What's more, this had taken a mere twenty-seven minutes of daily meditation. Other studies followed, suggesting significant changes could be achieved with as little as fifteen to twenty minutes. According to Lazar, fifty-year-old meditators have the same quantity of gray matter as people half their age.

Walking meditation combines the power of meditation with the benefits of movement and fresh air. And yet there's nothing new about it. Indeed, its roots lie in the sixth century BCE and the Buddha himself. Although the Buddha never hiked or "took a stroll," his was a life spent on foot. For fifty years the Buddha *walked* between towns, cities, and villages, conversing, teaching, and receiving alms. During the annual three-month monsoon retreat, his walking meditations are thought to have become more formalized, and the Pāli Canon—the first Buddhist scriptures to be communicated orally and eventually transcribed—highlights walking as one of the Buddha's four chosen "postures" for practicing mindfulness and achieving calm, clarity, and contentment.

But can walking meditation achieve the same impressive results as its traditionally seated counterpart? It appears so. One study found walking meditation reduced depression and stress symptoms while simultaneously increasing physical strength, flexibility, agility, balance, and cardiorespiratory endurance (a measure used by doctors to indicate our general level of health and fitness). The same study found that while *all* walking dramatically reduced inflammation and HDL cholesterol levels, only walking meditation lowered levels of cortisol, LDL cholesterol, and a protein called interleukin-6, implicated in inflammation and depression. Meanwhile, a 2019 study found that older women who practiced walking meditation also had better balance and coordination.

So how do we start? The Buddhist teacher Sylvia Boorstein recommends a thirty-minute slow walk, pointing out that while regular meditation follows the breath, walking meditation follows the rhythm of our steps. She recommends walking either inside or outside in a place that is "private and uncomplicated." The path must be at least ten to twenty feet long, with as few distractions as possible so that we can direct our full attention to our feet.

Close your eyes. Without moving, take a few long, deep breaths. Bring your attention to your body, starting with the soles of your feet, which should feel pleasantly rooted, moving up through your torso and arms to your head, then returning to your feet.

Open your eyes and begin walking, focusing on the lift and tread of your feet, the swing of your arms, or the sensation of your hands gently clasped behind your back. "Feel your whole body moving through space," says Boorstein. As your mind wanders, acknowledge the source of your distraction, then return to your body and the rhythmic lift and press of your feet. There's no need for any special gait or step. Move as slowly as you like, but keep returning attention to your feet, the deliberate roll of your soles against the ground, their continuous connection with the earth, the feeling of heaviness as you land, and the sense of lightness as you raise each leg.

Acknowledge the swing of your arms, the drifting scent of sap, the sound of birdsong, the way in which your breath comes and goes, the shift of pressure from one leg to the other, the rush of wind against your skin. Observe, acknowledge, but don't dwell on these things. Instead, return, always, to your feet and to your breath.

The Zen teacher Thich Nhat Hanh suggests experimenting with different patterns of breath, including lengthier exhalations where we "expel all the [stale] air from our lungs." By listening to our lungs, he explains, and playing with our breath-step patterns, we can transform how we breathe, improving our respiration and our circulation.

There is no right or wrong way to do walking meditation, no recommended speed, timing, posture, or location (although I'd suggest a path as smooth and straight as possible). The point is to use the physical process of walking to bring your attention entirely to the present. For many of us, the simple act of walking thrusts us into the moment, shutting down the endless chatter of our minds.

Walking meditation, however, involves a more focused attention on the beat of our feet, synchronizing this with our breath if we wish, as in Afghan walking (see Week 35: Walk Like a Nomad, p. 144). Like seated meditation, its walking counterpart trains our darting minds to be more attentive to the present. But it also keeps our limbs moving, our muscles working, and our blood flowing.

TIPS

WALKING MEDITATION CAN BE INCLUDED at the start or end of a walk, including a functional walk (to work or the supermarket, for example), making it particularly useful for those of us who are short of time.

Although Boorstein suggests thirty minutes, walking meditations can be as short as a few minutes and as slow or brisk as you prefer.

There are several walking meditation apps as well as YouTube tutorials for anyone wanting more guidance.

Prefer seated meditation? Try taking a walk immediately afterward. Studies suggest that combining seated meditation with a walk can achieve impressive results in those suffering from lower back pain or anxiety.

Alternatively, explore labyrinth walking, a centuries-old means of contemplation and relaxation. Find a labyrinth near you at World-Wide Labyrinth Locator (labyrinthlocator.com).

Walk Deep and Seek Out Fractals

A FEW YEARS AGO, THE writer and landscape consultant Tony Hiss went out to buy an iced coffee. His short walk to the bagel shop was an epiphany: "The familiar world outside immediately seemed—unexplored." Although he'd lived in New York City for most of his life, all at once "the familiar objects . . . seemed the most transformed . . . they now seemed charged with purpose . . . a story curled inside." Hiss's eye alighted on a blue mailbox, and instead of hurrying past, he let his mind play on how the mailbox came to be, the "great care and deliberation and . . . intelligence" that went into its design, manufacture, and locating. This moment of revelation—"awareness and attention had been intensified, reorganized, redeployed"—shifted the way in which he walked. He returned home "enriched and refreshed," but also with the germ of an idea: being in motion activates our capacity for adventure. Later, he coined the term *deep travel*. Arguably, his catalyzing walk to buy an iced coffee wasn't deep travel but *deep walking*.

A deep walk is, of necessity, a slow walk. Many of the walks in this book are of course methods of deep walking—ways of engaging our senses, our mind, and our spirit, as we move. When we observe birds, fungi, flowers, architecture, clouds, we deep walk. When we seek out sound, scent, silence, we deep walk. But there's another very simple way to transform a journey on foot into an adventure in deep walking: by seeking out fractals.

A fractal is a repeating pattern, often intricate, often identical—and often found in nature. Think of a snowflake, a fern, or an ocean wave, for example. Fractals are all around us, and looking at them is deeply pleasing. Indeed, physics professor Richard Taylor—who has been studying fractals for decades—believes that looking at fractal patterns "can induce staggering changes to the body" by reducing feelings of stress, improving cognitive skills, and heightening our ability to focus. Research using both EEGs (electroencephalograms) and fMRI (functional magnetic resonance imaging) confirms this: looking at fractals engages several parts of our brain, including the parahippocampus, which helps us process emotions as well as playing a significant role in spatial navigation and memory. Taylor's studies suggest that merely looking at fractal patterns can reduce our stress levels by 60 percent.

But not all fractals are equal, least of all when it comes to their ability to soothe us. Fractals are measured according to their complexity, or the rate at which the precise pattern reduces in size with each repetition. This is known as its fractal dimension, or D, and typically ranges from D1 to D2. Looser, larger, and less complex fractals score closer to D1 (like clouds or a flat landscape), while highly intricate, smaller, or tighter patterns score nearer to D2 (like the branching veins on a leaf or a dense forest). Taylor's studies show that we are most calmed by fractals that score at the low to mid range of complexity. When we look at fractals measuring between D1.3 and D1.5, our brains produce feel-good alpha brain waves: we are calmed and engaged, neither bored (D1) nor overwhelmed (D2).

More recently, a study in which young children were also exposed to fractals suggests that our appreciation of them begins before the age of three, leading researchers to speculate that we are hardwired to appreciate fractals, to find them deeply relaxing. Taylor thinks our innate love of fractals may derive from the way in which our eyes work—his experiments indicate that the human eye tracks using a fractal pattern of its own.

Fractals aren't in nature alone. They may be less abundant in cities, but look hard enough and fractals crop up (almost) everywhere—from church windows and the lichen on gravestones to flowers in the windows of florists and paintings in art galleries. (Art often makes use of fractals, as in Jackson Pollock's work, which has been fractally investigated in great depth by Taylor.) Nor do we need to peer at fractals for any length of time. According to Taylor, the exposure only has to be "environmental" . . . in other words, we can benefit merely from having fractals around us.

Looking for fractals is one of many ways in which we can deepen a walk. In my city—London—botanists organize weed walks through urban housing estates, which are as much about culture and history as wildflowers. Crumbling cemeteries are home to walking tours that include folklore, architecture, and the history of celebrities. Fungi walks involve hunting out toadstools and mushrooms from both hedgerows and the forgotten corners of urban parks. Many of these walks have fractals at their heart, but my point is this: search online and you'll find hundreds of remarkable individuals keen to share their vast knowledge, on foot, and often very inexpensively.

And here's the other thing about deep walking: it seems to activate and strengthen certain neurons in the brain. In 2021, Dutch neuroscientists discovered what they called a curiosity circuit in the brain of mice, a deeply buried region called the Zona Incerta. Experiments showed that the Zona Incerta lit up during "deep investigation" but remained inactive during "shallow investigations." Which is to suggest that deep walking might exercise our brains as much as it exercises our bodies.

Deep walking is not really about boosting brain cells. It's about changing our perception of walking, so that we no longer see it as dull, or as time *spent* getting somewhere, but as an unhurried opportunity for adventure, for encounters. As time *invested*. Hiss explained it like this: during "memorable trips, people . . . enter a different part of their own minds, and begin to make use of an awareness that has its own range of interests and concerns . . . [so] that the day itself seems more alive and full of possibility." I see it like this . . . In the cracks of pavement, in the fissured bark of fallen trees, under the thin skin of the earth, we can find entire universes.

TIPS

DEEP WALKING IS AT HEART attentive walking, so go alone or with a like-minded companion.

Deep walking is aided by knowledge, whether of geography, geology, architecture, history, fractals, or botany. Read up in advance, download an appropriate app, or find a knowledgeable walk leader.

Apps like Gesso can enliven city walks, as can organized walking tours, many of which now go quirkily beyond the usual and obvious tourist routes. Take a guided graffiti stroll in Berlin, an Underground River Walk in London, a walking seminar in Tokyo, a Women of Paris walking tour in Paris, or an "ethnic eating" tour in New York City.

Early mornings, when the streets are bright but empty, are ideal for deep urban walks.

Country walking with children? Encourage them to seek out as many fractals as possible.

Sketch the fractals you find (see Week 33: Sketch as You Walk, p. 135).

Share your own knowledge by transforming it into a walking route.

Afterword

AS *HOMO SAPIENS,* WE EVOLVED over eons to walk—all day, every day, bearing weight, through wind, rain, sun, and shadow, up and down hills, along rivers, through forests and over plains. We evolved in such a way that our 600 skeletal muscles were constantly moving. We evolved to have air in our lungs, scent in our nostrils, sun on our skin, breeze in our hair, sand and soil beneath our feet. And yet, as *Homo sapiens,* we also evolved to conserve our precious energy. Modern life panders to our innate desire to conserve energy—to do nothing. Never has it been easier to do so little, to move so infrequently. Never has it been more difficult to resist the alluring convenience of our electrified, pixelated age.

But resist we must. To preserve intact our collective body, brain, and soul, we need to be active and outdoors. Not all day but certainly every day. As human beings we are most fully alive when we move, when we encounter the world at a walking pace, when we step away from the quotidian comforts of home—and follow our senses.

This book is my love letter to walking. I hope it compels you to get up, get out, and get going, to relish the great privilege and richness of a life lived frequently on foot, and often in the wild, open air.

I'll leave the last word to my father, whose refusal to drive compelled me to walk, and who died as I was writing this book: "Move more gently. Consider the lightness of the feather. Follow the flight of the wren."

acknowledgments

MANY PEOPLE CONTRIBUTED TO THE MAKING OF THIS BOOK. In no particular order, I'd like to thank all those who gave so generously of their time and knowledge: Joanna Hall, Duncan Minshull, Dr. Tessa Pollard, Dr. Kate McLean, Lieutenant Liam O'Kelly, Subhadassie, Ellen Cooper de Groote, Dr. Helen Cox, Dr. Charlotte Megeney, the British Pilgrimage Trust, Brian Prendergast, Roy Vickery, Martin Christie, the Sussex Ornithological Society, and walking artist Geraldine van Heemstra. I'd like to thank all the researchers whose books, podcasts, studies, and reports I have repeatedly leaned on—and without whose tireless work this book would not exist. Any mistakes are mine and mine alone.

Thank you to all the people who helped me turn an idea into this book: my hardworking agents, Rachel Mills in London and Stuart Krichevsky in New York; my wonderful editors and their teams—Michelle Howry, with Sally Kim, Ashley Hewlett, Colleen Nuccio, Ashley Di Dio, Maija Baldauf, Lorie Pagnozzi, and the rest of the team at Putnam; and Rowan Yapp with Lauren Whybrow at Bloomsbury. And thank you to Alexis Seabrook for the beautiful illustrations in this book.

A huge thank-you to all the friends and companions who have walked with me over the years: you know who you are. Most of all, I thank my family, who have walked beside me across dozens of cities, up and down mountains, in driving rain and stubborn heat, through starlit fields and darkest forests, on litter picks, forages, dawn strolls, and barefoot yomps, often lost but always—eventually—found.

notes

Introduction

xv   average American walked 1.4 miles: Bill Bryson, *A Walk in the Woods* (Broadway Books, 1998).

xvi   militarily *rucked*: Rucking is a military term for brisk walking with a pack, often for long distance. See more in Week 36: Hike with a Pack, p. 148.

xvii   4 million premature deaths: Tessa Strain, Søren Brage, et al., "Use of the prevented fraction for the population to determine deaths averted by existing prevalence of physical activity: A descriptive study," *The Lancet Global Health* 8, no. 7 (2020): e920—e930.

xvii   8 million deaths a year: Peter Walker, *The Miracle Pill: Why a Sedentary World Is Getting It All Wrong* (Simon & Schuster, 2021).

xvii   thirty-five chronic diseases: Sean L. McGee and Mark Hargreaves, "Exercise adaptations: Molecular mechanisms and potential targets for therapeutic benefit," *Nature Reviews Endocrinology* 16 (2020): 495–505.

xvii   more resistant to disease: Joji Kusuyama, Ana Barbara Alves-Wagner, et al., "Effects of maternal and paternal exercise on offspring metabolism," *Nature Metabolism* 2 (2020): 858–72.

xvii   babies' lifelong risk: Johan E. Harris, Kelsey M. Pinckard, et al., "Exercise-induced 3′-sialyllactose in breast milk is a critical mediator to improve metabolic health and cardiac function in mouse offspring," *Nature Metabolism* 2, no. 8 (2020): 678–87.

Week 1: Walk in the Cold

5   "whistling winds and driving snows": Kerri Andrews, *Wanderers: A History of Women Walking* (Reaktion Books, 2020).

5   living in the Arctic Circle: Christiane Ritter, *A Woman in the Polar Night* (Greystone Books, 2010; originally published 1938).

5   "paradise": Alexandra David-Néel, *My Journey to Lhasa* (Dead Authors Society, 2020; originally published 1927), p. 118.

6   "headaches and cancerous tumors": S. M. Cooper and R. P. R. Dawber, "The history of cryosurgery," *Journal of the Royal Society of Medicine* 94, no. 4 (April 2001): 196–201.

6   complexities of cold: R. Imamura, M. Funatsu, et al., "Effects of wearing long- and mini-skirts for a year on subcutaneous fat thickness and body circumference," paper presented at the IXth Conference on Environmental Ergonomics, Aachen (Shaker Verlag, 2000).

6   remarkable truth about brown fat: Carol Cruzan Morton, "Research on Brown Fat Heats Up," Harvard Medical School News & Research, May 1, 2009, https://hms .harvard.edu/news/research-brown-fat-heats.

7   and coronary artery disease: Tobias Becher, Srikanth Palanisamy, et al., "Brown adipose tissue is associated with cardiometabolic health," *Nature Medicine* 27 (January 4, 2021): 58–65.

7   reflecting a 2012 study: Adrian F. Ward, "Winter Wakes Up Your Mind—and Warm Weather Makes It Harder to Think Straight," *Scientific American*, February 12, 2013, https://www.scientificamerican.com/article/warm-weather-makes-it-hard-think-straight/.

8   peripheral vision: Eliran Halali, Nachshon Meiran, and Idit Shalev, "Keep it cool: Temperature priming effect on cognitive control," *Psychological Research* 81, no. 2 (March 2017): 343–54.

8   green-gold spring: Ernest Bielinis et al., "The effect of winter forest bathing on psychological relaxation of young Polish adults," *Urban Forestry & Urban Greening* 29 (January 2018): 276–83.

8   2018 report from the University of Luxembourg: Manuela Jungmann, Shervin Vencatachellum, et al., "Effects of cold stimulation on cardiac-vagal activation in healthy participants: Randomized controlled trial," *JMIR Formative Research* 2, no. 2 (2018): e10257.

8   bodies work more efficiently: "The Wonders of Winter Workouts," Harvard Men's Health Watch, December 1, 2018, https://www.health.harvard.edu/staying-healthy/the-wonders-of-winter-workouts.

8   Wouter van Marken Lichtenbelt: Morton, "Research on Brown Fat Heats Up."

9   improving respiratory symptoms: Johanna Prossegger et al., "Winter exercise reduces allergic airway inflammation: A randomized controlled study." *International Journal of Environmental Research and Public Health* 16, no. 11 (June 2019): 2040; and Johanna Freidl et al. "Winter exercise and speleotherapy for allergy and asthma: A randomized controlled clinical trial," *Journal of Clinical Medicine* 9, no. 10 (2020): 3311, for example. But check with your doctor first.

9   Harvard Medical School: Morton, "Research on Brown Fat Heats Up."

Week 2: Improve Your Gait

10   neurodegenerative conditions: Frederico Pieruccini-Faria, Sandra E. Black, et al., "Gait variability across neurodegenerative and cognitive disorders: Results from the Canadian Consortium of Neurodegeneration in Aging (CCNA) and the Gait

and Brain Study." *Alzheimer's & Dementia*, February 16, 2021, DOI: 10:1002/alz.12298.

11 walk as their bodies intended: Joanna Hall's WalkActive program can be found online at https://joannahallwalkactive.com/ or on YouTube.

12 improved skeletal alignment: "Walk this way: LSBU research spearheads nationwide 'Walkactive' campaign," LSBU, June 6, 2014, https://www.lsbu.ac.uk/about-us/news/walk-this-way-lsbu-research-spearheads-nationwide-walkactive-campaign.

12 "shorter steps but more of them": "Walk This Way to Protect Your Neck," Harvard Medical School, Staying Healthy, September 24, 2020, https://www.health.harvard.edu/staying-healthy/walk-this-way-to-protect-your-neck.

13 "important health conditions": Carlos A. Celis Morales et al., "Walking pace is associated with lower risk of all-cause and cause-specific mortality," *Medicine and Science in Sports and Exercise* 51, no. 3 (March 2019): 472–80.

13 improving mood: Kannin B. Osei-Tutu and Phil D. Campagna, "The effects of short- vs. long-bout exercise on mood, VO_{2max}, and percent body fat," *Preventive Medicine* 40, no. 1 (January 2005): 92–98.

Week 3: Walk, Smile, Greet, Repeat

16 feeling more upbeat: "When you're smiling, the whole world really does smile with you," University of South Australia, August 12, 2020, https://www.unisa.edu.au/Media-Center/Releases/2020/when-youre-smiling-the-whole-world-really-does-smile-with-you/.

16 those who were ignored: Eric D. Wesselmann, Florencia D. Cardoso, et al., "To be looked at as though air: Civil attention matters," *Psychological Science* 23, no. 2 (2012): 166–68.

17 believe in themselves: "Body posture affects confidence in your own thoughts, study finds," *Science Daily*, October 5, 2009, https://www.sciencedaily.com/releases/2009/10/091005111627.htm.

17 slumped students: Erik Peper, Richard Harvey, et al., "Do better in math: How your body posture may change stereotype threat response," *NeuroRegulation* 5, no. 2 (2018): 67–74.

17 study after study: See, for instance, "Mental health statistics: Relationships and community," Mental Health Foundation, https://www.mentalhealth.org.uk/statistics/mental-health-statistics-relationships-and-community.

Week 4: Just One Slow Walk

19 learn, focus, and remember: "The human milk oligosaccharide, 3'SL, in pre-weaning milk influences attention, learning and memory later in life," Nestlé Nutrition Institute, May 14, 2020, https://www.nestlenutrition-institute.org/news/article/2020/05/14/the-human-milk-oligosaccharide-3-sl-in-pre-weaning-milk-influences-attention-learning-and-memory-later-in-life.

19 mothers' milk: Johan E. Harris, Kelsey M. Pinckard, et al., "Exercise-induced 3'-sialyllactose in breast milk is a critical mediator to improve metabolic health and

cardiac function in mouse offspring," *Nature Metabolism* 2, no. 8 (2020): 678–87.

19   "a substantially lower risk of death": "Physical activity at any intensity linked to lower risk of early death," *BMJ, Science Daily,* August 21, 2019, https://www.bmj .com/company/newsroom/physical-activity-at-any-intensity-linked-to-lower- risk-of-early-death/.

20   "Light physical activity can help": Saurabh S. Thosar, Sylvanna L. Bielko, et al., "Effect of prolonged sitting and breaks in sitting time on endothelial function," *Medicine & Science in Sports & Exercise* 47, no. 4 (April 2015): 843–49.

20   time spent sitting: Bernard M. F. M. Duvivier, Nicolaas Schaper, et al., "Minimal intensity physical activity (standing and walking) of longer duration improves insulin action and plasma lipids more than shorter periods of moderate to vigorous exercise (cycling) in sedentary subjects when energy expenditure is comparable," *PLoS One* 8, no. 2 (2013): e55542.

20   up to 25 percent: Raymond C. Browning and Rodger Kram, "Energetic cost and preferred speed of walking in obese vs. normal weight women," *Obesity* 13, no. 5 (2005): 891–99.

20   "whether you live or die": "Step Up Your Walking Game," Harvard Medical School Heart Health, July 1, 2020, https://www.health.harvard.edu/heart-health /step-up-your-walking-game.

21   neuroradiologist: A neuroradiologist is a radiologist specializing in the central nervous system—the brain, spinal cord, neck, and head.

21   breathing: Jacqueline Brenner, Suzanne LeBlang, et al., "Mindfulness with paced breathing reduces blood pressure," *Medical Hypotheses* 142 (September 2020): 109780.

21   vagus nerve: The intricate and complex vagus nerve is one of twelve pairs of cranial nerves carrying information from various body parts to our brain. It plays a vital role in our ability to relax and digest, among other things.

21   as research intensifies: There have been many reports; this is just one: Xiao Wu et al., "Exposure to air pollution and COVID-19 mortality in the United States: A nationwide cross-sectional study," *Science Advances* 6, no. 45 (November 4, 2020): eabd4049.

21   less than two hours a week: Mathew P. White, Ian Alcock, et al., "Spending at least 120 minutes a week in nature is associated with good health and wellbeing," *Nature Scientific Reports* 9 (2019): article number 7730.

21   "walk of twenty miles": C. C. Vyvyan, *Roots and Stars* (The Country Book Club, 1963).

Week 5: Breathe as You Walk

23   survive for longer: For more on the process of cellular aging, see Annabel Streets and Susan Saunders, *The Age-Well Project: Easy Ways to a Longer, Healthier, Happier Life* (Piatkus, 2019).

24   fighting back: One of the many studies exploring this is Jan Martel, Yun-Fei Ko, et al., "Could nasal nitric oxide help to mitigate the severity of COVID-19?" *Microbes and Infection* 22, no. 4 (May–June 2020): 168–171.

24   "into our lungs": Laura Hood, "The right way to breathe during the coronavirus pandemic," *The Conversation*, June 19, 2020, https://theconversation.com/the-right-way-to-breathe-during-the-coronavirus-pandemic-140695.

24   through the nose: George M. Dallam, Steve R. McClaren, et al., "Effect of nasal versus oral breathing on VO2max and physiological economy in recreational runners following an extended period spent using nasally restricted breathing," *International Journal of Kinesiology & Sports Science* 6, no. 2 (2018): 22–29.

24   bad breath: James Nestor, *Breath: The Lost Science of a New Art* (Penguin, 2020).

25   nitric oxide: Eddie Weitzberg and Jon O. N. Lundberg, "Humming greatly increases nasal nitric oxide," *American Journal of Respiratory and Critical Care Medicine* 166, no. 2 (2002): 144–45.

Week 6: Take a Muddy Walk

26   tuberculosis: Greg St. Martin, "Newly discovered antibiotic kills pathogens without resistance," News at Northeastern, January 7, 2015, News@Northeastern, https://news.northeastern.edu/2015/01/07/kim-lewis-teixobactin-nature-paper/.

27   consume the bacterium: Debora Mackenzie, "Eat bacteria to boost brain power," May 27, 2010, *New Scientist*, https://www.newscientist.com/article/dn18967-eat-bacteria-to-boost-brain-power/.

27   boost their immune systems: M. E. R. O'Brien, H. Anderson, et al., "SRL172 (killed Mycobacterium vaccae) in addition to standard chemotherapy improves quality of life without affecting survival, in patients with advanced non-small-cell lung cancer: Phase III results," *Annals of Oncology* 15, no. 6 (June 2004): 906–14.

27   "learn new tasks": Anne Cissel, "It's in the dirt! Bacteria in soil may make us happier, smarter," National Wildlife Federation, March 9, 2011, https://blog.nwf.org/2011/03/its-in-the-dirt-bacteria-in-soil-may-make-us-happier-smarter/.

27   bacterium: The bacterium is called *Kineothrix alysoides*.

28   mental health: Craig Liddicoat, Harrison Sydnor, et al., "Naturally-diverse airborne environmental microbial exposures modulate the gut microbiome and may provide anxiolytic benefits in mice," *Science of the Total Environment* 701 (January 20, 2020): 134684.

28   living environment: Interview with the author, September 18, 2020.

29   toxic compounds into the environment: Kristen Coyne, "FSU researchers find sun and rain transform asphalt binder into potentially toxic compounds," Florida State University News, July 13, 2020, https://news.fsu.edu/news/science-technology/2020/07/13/fsu-researchers-find-sun-and-rain-transform-asphalt-binder-into-potentially-toxic-compounds/.

Week 7: Take a Twelve-Minute Walk

30 a (very short) walk: Matthew Nayor, Ravi V. Shah, et al., "Metabolic architecture of acute exercise response in middle-aged adults in the community," *Circulation* 142, no. 20 (September 15, 2020): 1905–24.

31 liver disease and diabetes: dimethylguanidino valeric acid (DMGV).

31 fat stores: 1-methylnicotinamide.

31 *Men's Health* magazine: Edward Cooper, "Just 12 Minutes of Exercise Offers Huge Benefits, Harvard-Affiliated Study Finds," *Men's Health*, December 12, 2020. https://www.menshealth.com/uk/health/a34845423/small-workouts-harvard-study-health/.

31 particularly for women: Michael J. Wheeler et al., "Effect of Morning Exercise With or Without Breaks in Prolonged Sitting on Blood Pressure in Older Overweight/Obese Adults," *Hypertension* 73, no. 4 (2019): 859–67.

Week 8: Walk with Vista Vision

34 organized and stored: This is, of necessity, a very abbreviated discussion of how EMDR works. See http://www.emdr.com/ for more information.

34 process, store, and retrieve: D. Eric Chamberlin, "The Predictive Processing Model of EMDR," *Frontiers in Psychology* 10 (October 4, 2019): 2267.

34 panoramic vision: See Huberman Lab, Department of Neurobiology at Stanford University, http://www.hubermanlab.com/index.html.

35 walking helps restore it: Liyu Cao, Barbara Händel, "Walking Enhances Peripheral Visual Processing in Humans," *PLoS Biol* 17, no. 10 (2019): e3000511.

35 than if we look around: Shana Cole, Matthew Riccio, Emily Balcetis. "Focused and Fired Up: Narrowed Attention Produces Perceived Proximity and Increases Goal-Relevant Action," *Motivation and Emotion* 38 (2014): 815–22.

35 "How new it has become!": Nan Shepherd, *The Living Mountain* (Canongate, 2019; first published 1977).

Week 9: Take a Windy Walk

36 "natural experience": Douglas Mawson, *The Home of the Blizzard*, vol. 1, 1915.

37 "prickles of apprehension": Lyall Watson, *Heaven's Breath: A Natural History of the Wind* (Hodder & Stoughton, 1984).

37 in our DNA: Theo A. Klimstra, Tom Frijns, et al., "Come rain or come shine: Individual differences in how weather affects mood," *Emotion* 11, no. 6 (2011): 1495–99.

37 lowered the mood of others: Dick Ettema et al., "Season and Weather Effects on Travel-Related Mood and Travel Satisfaction," *Frontiers in Psychology* 8 (2017): 140.

37 than men: Marie Connolly, "Some Like It Mild and Not Too Wet: The Influence of Weather on Subjective Well-Being," *Journal of Happiness Studies* 14 (2013): 457–73.

38 seeds of discontent: Annabel Abbs, *Windswept: Walking the Paths of Trailblazing Women* (Portland: Tin House, 2020).

Week 10: Walk Within an Hour of Waking

40 "for my work": Kerri Andrews, *Wanderers: A History of Women Walking* (London: Reaktion Books, 2020), 135.

41 sleep soundly: A. Panzer, "Depression or cancer: the choice between serotonin or melatonin?" *Medical Hypotheses* 50, no. 5 (1998): 385–87.

41 role our eyes play: Yoshimasa Oyama, Colleen M. Bartman, et al., "Intense light-mediated circadian cardioprotection via transcriptional reprogramming of the endothelium," *Cell Reports* 28, no. 6 (2019): 1471–84.e11.

42 pictures of food: Bliss Hanlon, Michael J. Larson, et al., "Neural response to pictures of food after exercise in normal-weight and obese women," *Medicine & Science in Sports & Exercise* 44, no. 10 (2012): 1864–70.

42 control food intake: Jae Hoon Jeong, Dong Kun Lee, et al., "Activation of temperature-sensitive TRPV1-like receptors in ARC POMC neurons reduces food intake," *PLoS Biology* 16, no. 4 (April 24, 2018): e2004399.

42 effects on human beings: Anders B. Klein, Trine S. Nicolaisen, et al., "Pharmacological but not physiological GDF15 suppresses feeding and the motivation to exercise," *Nature Communications* 12 (2021), article no. 1041.

43 other than eight P.M.: Jun Wang and Shu-hua Li, "Changes in negative air ions concentration under different light intensities and development of a model to relate light intensity to directional change," *Journal of Environmental Management* 90, no. 8 (2009): 2746–54.

43 later in the day: James Martin, "Dawn Chorus: Why Do Birds Sing in the Morning?" Woodland Trust, April 19, 2019, https://www.woodlandtrust.org.uk /blog/2019/04/dawn-chorus/#:~:text=Why%20do%20birds%20sing% 20so,would%20later%20in%20the%20day.

43 up to four hours: "Exposure to trees, the sky and birdsong in cities beneficial for mental wellbeing," King's College London News Centre, January 16, 2018, https://www.kcl.ac.uk/news/spotlight/exposure-to-trees-the-sky-and-birdsong-in-cities-beneficial-for-mental-wellbeing.

Week 11: Take a City Smell Walk

45 smellscapes: Sensory Maps: Research, analysis & design of Sensory Maps by Kate McLean, http://sensorymaps.blogspot.com/.

45 every hour: Sensory Maps: Research, analysis & design of Sensory Maps by Kate McLean, http://sensorymaps.blogspot.com/.

45 each of our nostrils: Xi Li and Forshing Lui, "Anosmia," StatPearls, March 24, 2021, https://www.ncbi.nlm.nih.gov/books/NBK482152/.

45 heart disease: Victoria Van Regemorter, Thomas Hummel, et al., "Mechanisms linking olfactory impairment and risk of mortality," *Frontiers in Neuroscience* 14 (February 21, 2020): 140.

45 depression and anxiety: Marlene M. Speth, Thirza Singer-Cornelius, et al., "Mood, anxiety and olfactory dysfunction in COVID-19: Evidence of central nervous system involvement?" *Laryngoscope* 130, no. 11 (2020): 2520–25.

45   fear and sadness: Shirin Masjedi, Laurence J. Zwiebel, and Todd D. Giorgio, "Olfactory receptor gene abundance in invasive breast carcinoma," *Scientific Reports* 9, article no. 13736 (2019).

46   thickness in several brain areas: Syrina Al Aïn, Daphnée Poupon, et al., "Smell training improves olfactory function and alters brain structure," *Neuroimage* 189 (2019): 45–54.

Week 12: Walk in the Rain

48   "as good as drunk": Nan Shepherd, *The Living Mountain* (Canongate, 2019; first published 1977).

49   "perfume of the earth": Cynthia Barnett, "Making Perfume from the Rain," *The Atlantic*, April 22, 2015, https://www.theatlantic.com/international/archive/2015/04/making-perfume-from-the-rain/391011/.

49   after a downpour: Jennifer Chu, "Can rain clean the atmosphere?" MIT News Office, August 28, 2015, http://news.mit.edu/2015/rain-drops-attract-aerosols-clean-air-0828.

49   particals of PM2.5: PM2.5 are particles of air pollution 100 times thinner than a human hair and able to travel across the blood-brain barrier as well as deep into the lungs. Breathing in these microscopic particles has been linked to numerous health conditions from COVID-19 to heart disease, dementia, lung cancer, and asthma. For more information see https://www.pnas.org/content/117/25/13856.

50   surge of dopamine: Nico Bunzeck and Emrah Düzel, "Absolute coding of stimulus novelty in the human substantia nigra/VTA," *Neuron* 51, no. 3 (August 3, 2006): 369–79.

50   exercise in the rain: R. Ito, M. Nakano, et al., "Effects of rain on energy metabolism while running in a cold environment," *International Journal of Sports Medicine* 34, no. 8 (2013): 707–11.

Week 13: Take a Walk-Dance or a Dance-Walk

51   to write a book: Will Kemp, *Kemps nine daies wonder. Performed in a daunce from London to Norwich . . .* written by himself, printed 1600, held at the Bodleian Library, University of Oxford.

51   one day faster: "Morris man arrives in Norwich after 120-mile dance," *Eastern Daily Press*, February 23, 2011, https://www.edp24.co.uk/news/morris-man-arrives-in-norwich-after-120-mile-dance-471434.

52   more joyful lives: René T. Proyer, Fabian Gander, et al., "Can playfulness be stimulated? A randomised placebo-controlled online playfulness intervention study on effects on trait playfulness, well-being, and depression," *Applied Psychology: Health and Well-Being* 13, no. 1 (February 2021): 129–51.

52   larger brains: Robert Sanders, "Marian Diamond, known for studies of Einstein's brain, dies at 90," Berkeley News, July 28, 2017, https://news.berkeley.edu/2017/07/28/marian-diamond-known-for-studies-of-einsteins-brain-dies-at-90/.

53 more ideas than normal walkers: Michael L. Slepian and Nalini Ambady, "Fluid movement and creativity," *Journal of Experimental Psychology: General* 141, no. 4 (2012): 625–29.

53 McMaster University: Ana Kovakevic, Barbara Fenesi, et al., "The effects of aerobic exercise intensity on memory in older adults," *Applied Physiology, Nutrition and Metabolism* 45, no. 6 (June 2020): 591–600.

53 Miranda Hart style: See "Miranda—Galloping" on YouTube: https://www .youtube.com/watch?v=pmKtC8_4_wM.

Week 14: Walk with Your Ears

55 natural sounds decreased anxiety: Brent A. Bauer, Susanne A. Cutshall, et al., "Effect of the combination of music and nature sounds on pain and anxiety in cardiac surgical patients: a randomized study," *Alternative Therapies in Health and Medicine* 17, no. 4 (2011): 16–23.

55 classical music: Myriam Verena Thoma, Ricarda Mewes, and Urs M. Nater, "Preliminary evidence: The stress-reducing effect of listening to water sounds depends on somatic complaints," *Medicine* (*Baltimore*) 97, no. 8 (2018): e9851.

56 natural sounds: Cassandra D. Gould van Praag, Sarah N. Garfinkel, et al., "Mind-wandering and alterations to default mode network connectivity when listening to naturalistic versus artificial sounds," *Nature: Scientific Reports* 7, article no. 45273 (2017).

56 a million years of healthy life: *Burden of Disease from Environmental Noise— Quantification of Healthy Life Years Lost in Europe*, WHO Regional Office for Europe (Copenhagen, 2011).

57 birdsong made them feel happy: "Woodland sounds boost wellbeing according to new study," National Trust, September 12, 2019, https://www.nationaltrust.org .uk/press-release/woodland-sounds-boost-wellbeing-according-to-new-study.

57 listening to the real thing—outside: Anette Kjellgren, Hanne Buhrkall, "A Comparison of the Restorative Effect of a Natural Environment with That of a Simulated Natural Environment," *Journal of Environmental Psychology* 30, no. 4 (2010): 464–72.

Week 15: Walk Alone

59 "the great world beating": Clara Vyvyan, *Journey Up the Years* (Peter Owen, 1966).

60 "silence of the morning": William Hazlitt, "On Going a Journey," 1822, quoted in Duncan Minshull, ed., *While Wandering: A Walking Companion* (Vintage, 2014).

60 essential as exercise or healthy eating: Jack Fong, "A View from Sociology: The Role of Solitude in Transcending Social Crises—New Possibilities for Existential Sociology," from Robert J. Coplan and Julie C. Bowker, eds., *The Handbook of Solitude* (John Wiley, 2013), 499–516.

60 "his highest potential": Anthony Storr, *Solitude: A Return to the Self* (HarperCollins, 1997).

60   greater feelings of satisfaction: R. Larson and M. Lee, "The capacity to be alone as a stress buffer," *Journal of Social Psychology* 136, no. 1 (1996): 5–16.

60   quality of our relationships: Adital Ben-Ari, "Rethinking closeness and distance in intimate relationships: Are they really two opposites?" *Journal of Family Issues* 33, no. 3 (2012): 391–412.

60   "without great solitude": Thuy-Vy T. Nguyen, Richard M. Ryan, and Edward L. Dec, "Solitude as an approach to affective self-regulation," *Personality and Social Psychology Bulletin* 44, no. 1 (2018): 92–106.

61   "compass across the hills": Dorothy Pilley, *Climbing Days* (Quinn Press, 2011; originally published 1935).

61   "self-strengthening": See, for instance, Matthew H. Bowker, "A View from Political Theory: Desire, Subjectivity, and Pseudo-Solitude," from Robert J. Coplan and Julie C. Bowker, eds., *The Handbook of Solitude* (John Wiley, 2013), 539–56.

61   "deeper than memory": Pilley, *Climbing Days*.

61   when we walk alone: Lia Noar and Ofra Mayseless, "How personal transformation occurs following a single peak experience in nature: A phenomenological account," *Journal of Humanistic Psychology* 60, no. 6 (2017): 1–24.

62   build from there: Matthew Bowker, "Interview on the Stigmatisation of Solitude," September 9, 2018, https://matthewhbowker.com/2018/09/09/interview-on-the-stigmatisation-of-solitude-elle-magazine-uk/.

Week 16: Pick Up Litter as You Walk

63   "it's really rewarding": Olivia Mukerjea, "'Litter picking has saved their life': How doing an hour of litter picking can improve your mental health," Salford Now, October 13, 2020, http://www.salfordnow.co.uk/2020/10/13/litter-picking-has-saved-their-life-how-doing-an-hour-of-litter-picking-can-improve-your-mental-health/.

64   meaning and purpose: Kayleigh J. Wyles, Sabine Pahl, et al., "Can beach cleans do more than clean-up litter? Comparing beach cleans to other coastal activities," *Environment and Behavior* 49, no. 5 (2017): 509–35.

65   reduced rates of mortality: Rodlescia S. Sneed and Sheldon Cohen, "A prospective study of volunteerism and hypertension risk in older adults," *Psychology and Aging* 28, no. 2 (2013): 578–86.

65   nonvolunteering counterparts: Hayley Guiney and Liana Machado, "Volunteering in the community: Potential benefits for cognitive aging," *Journals of Gerontology, Series B: Psychological Sciences and Social Sciences* 73, no. 3 (2018): 399–408.

66   royal family can pick up litter: Hannah Furness, "Princes William and Harry reveal how they got teased after their father used to take them on litter-picking holiday," *Telegraph*, November 4, 2018, https://www.telegraph.co.uk/news/2018/11/04/princes-william-harry-reveal-got-teased-father-used-take-litter/.

Week 17: Follow a River

67   her happiness fully restored: Annabel Abbs, *Windswept: Walking the Paths of Trailblazing Women* (Two Roads, 2021).

67 "near the river": Kerri Andrews, *Wanderers: A History of Women Walking* (Reaktion Books, 2020).

68 passing through it: C. L. E. Rohde and A. D. Kendle, "Human well-being, natural landscapes and wildlife in urban areas: a review," English Nature Science Reports, January 1, 1994, http://publications.naturalengland.org.uk/publication/2320898.

68 less depression: Sebastian Völker and Thomas Kistermann, "The impact of blue space on human health and well-being—Salutogenetic health effects of inland surface waters: a review," *International Journal of Hygiene and Environmental Health* 214, no. 6 (November 2011): 449–460.

68 music or silence: Myriam Verena Thoma, Ricarda Mewes, and Urs M. Nater, "Preliminary evidence: The stress-reducing effect of listening to water sounds depends on somatic complaints," *Medicine (Baltimore)* 97, no. 8 (February 2018): e9851.

68 attention restoration theory: This idea originates in the 1989 book *Experience of Nature* by Stephen and Rachel Kaplan and proposes that exposure to nature helps people improve focus and ability to concentrate.

70 delay the onset of dementia: "How cold water swimming could slow the onset of dementia," BBC News: Health, October 19, 2020, https://www.bbc.co.uk/news/av/health-54600555.

Week 18: Walk with a Dog

71 "my guard in my long solitary walks": Mary Eyre, *A Lady's Walks in the South of France* (1865).

72 "the Lassie effect": C. Westgarth, M. Knuiman, and H. E. Christian, "Understanding how dogs encourage and motivate walking: Cross-sectional findings from RESIDE," *BMC Public Health* 16, no. 1 (2016): 1019.

72 in better health: Bruce Headey and Markus M. Grabka, "Pets and human health in Germany and Australia: National longitudinal results," *Social Indicators Research* 80 (2007): 297–311.

72 a result of their extra walking: Quoted in Annabel Streets and Susan Saunders, *The Age-Well Project: Easy Ways to a Longer, Healthier, Happier Life* (Piatkus, 2019).

73 therapy dogs reduced stress and anxiety: Chia-Chun Tsai, Erika Friedmann, and Sue A. Thomas, "The effect of animal-assisted therapy on stress responses in hospitalized children," *Anthrozoös* 23, no. 3 (2010): 245–58.

73 if a rehabilitation dog was involved: Lynda Rondeau, Hélène Corriveau, et al., "Effectiveness of a rehabilitation dog in fostering gait retraining for adults with a recent stroke: A multiple single-case study," *NeuroRehabilitation* 27, no. 2 (2010): 155–63.

73 "Are pets the new probiotic?": Richard Schiffman, "Are Pets the New Probiotic?" *New York Times*, June 6, 2017.

73 dog owners have higher self-esteem: Claudia Schultz, Hans-Helmut König, and André Hajek, "Differences in self-esteem between cat owners, dog owners, and individuals without pets," *Frontiers in Veterinary Science* 7 (September 2, 2020): 552.

74 helping children's social-emotional development: Elizabeth J. Wenden, Leanne Lester, et al., "The relationship between dog ownership, dog play, family dog walking, and preschooler social-emotional development: Findings from the PLAYCE observational study," *Pediatric Research* 89, no. 4 (2021): 1013–19.

Week 19: Amble amid Trees

76 high blood pressure, and stress: Caoimhe Twohig-Bennett and Andy Jones, "The health benefits of the great outdoors: A systematic review and meta-analysis of greenspace exposure and health outcomes," *Environmental Research* 166 (2018): 628–37.

76 immediate improvements in well-being after walking among trees: Liisa Tyrväinen, Ann Ojala, et al., "Health and well-being from forests—experience from Finnish research [article in French]," *Santé publique* (Vandoeuvre-les-Nancy, France), May 13, 2019: 249–56.

76 reducing inflammation: Katherine Ka-Yin Yau and Alice Yuen Loke, "Effects of forest bathing on pre-hypertensive and hypertensive adults: A review of the literature," *Environmental Health and Preventive Medicine* 25 (2020): 23.

76 people living in leafy neighborhoods remained mentally sharper: "Largest Study Ever Finds That Urban Green Space Can Prevent Premature Deaths," Barcelona Institute for Global Health, November 21, 2019, https://www.eurekalert.org /pub_releases/2019-11/bifg-lse111919.php.

77 what makes a tree so therapeutic: Ming Kuo et al., "Greening for academic achievement: Prioritizing what to plant and where," *Landscape and Urban Planning* 206 (February 2021): 103962.

77 more effective than antidepressants: Qing Li, *Shinrin-Yoku: The Art and Science of Forest Bathing* (Penguin, 2018).

78 "parallel changes in their immune systems": Marja I. Roslund, Riikka Puhakka, et al., "Biodiversity intervention enhances immune regulation and health-associated commensal microbiota among daycare children," *Science Advances* 6, no. 42 (October 2020): eaba2578.

79 "three days in woodland increased NK cells by 50 percent": Qing Li, *Shinrin-Yoku*.

79 Take a weekly walk if possible: Denise Mitten, Jillisa R. Overholt, et al., "Hiking: A low-cost, accessible intervention to promote health benefits," *American Journal of Lifestyle Medicine* 12, no. 4 (2018).

Week 20: Walk to Remember

80 more marked among the children: Sabine Schaefer et al., "Cognitive performance is improved while walking: Differences in cognitive-sensorimotor couplings between children and young adults," *European Journal of Developmental Psychology* 7, no. 3 (2010): 371–89.

80 similar experiment was taking place in the United States: Carlos R. Salas, Katsumi Minakata, and William L. Kelemen, "Walking before study enhances free recall

but not judgment-of-learning magnitude," *Journal of Cognitive Psychology* 23, no. 4 (2011): 507–13.

81   improved associative memory: Associative memory is commonly described as the ability to learn and remember the relationship between unrelated items, like faces and names, for example.

82   mnemonic time travel effect: Aleksandar Aksentijevic, Kaz R. Brandt, et al., "It takes me back: The mnemonic time-travel effect," *Cognition* 182 (2018): 242–50.

83   greater emotional resilience: Megan E. Speer and Mauricio R. Delgado, "Reminiscing about positive memories buffers acute stress responses," *Nature Human Behavior* 1, no. 5 (2017): 0093; and "Recalling positive events and experiences can help protect young people against depression in later life," Cambridge Neuroscience, https://www.neuroscience.cam.ac.uk/news/article.php?permalink=0677198f2c.

83   cutting their risk of memory loss in half: K. I. Erickson, C. A. Raji, et al., "Physical activity predicts gray matter volume in late adulthood: The Cardiovascular Health Study," *Neurology* 75, no. 16 (October 19, 2010): 1415–22.

83   slow the path of Alzheimer's: Tsubasa Tomoto, Jie Liu, et al., "One-year aerobic exercise reduced carotid arterial stiffness and increased cerebral blood flow in amnestic mild cognitive impairment," *Journal of Alzheimer's Disease* 80, no. 2 (2021): 841–53.

83   lasted for an hour: Y. K. Chang, J. D. Labban, et al., "The effects of acute exercise on cognitive performance: A meta-analysis," *Brain Research* 1453 (May 9, 2012): 87–101.

83   Walking is the perfect intensity: Roy David Samuel, Ofir Zavdy, et al., "The effects of maximal intensity exercise on cognitive performance in children," *Journal of Human Kinetics* 57 (June 2017): 85–96.

Week 21: Exercise Your Curiosity Muscle—Walk a Ley Line

85   two books: Alfred Watkins, *Early British Trackways* (1921), and *The Old Straight Track* (1925).

85   long-gone funeral paths: Danny Sullivan, *Ley Lines—A Comprehensive Guide to Alignments* (Green Magic, 2004).

86   "retain any kind of information": Matthias J. Gruber, Maureen Ritchey, et al., "Post-learning hippocampal dynamics promote preferential retention of rewarding events," *Neuron* 89, no. 5 (March 2, 2016): 1110–20.

86   "meaning and life-satisfaction": Todd B. Kashdan and Michael F. Steger, "Curiosity and pathways to well-being and meaning in life: Traits, states, and everyday behaviors," *Motivation & Emotion* 31 (2007): 159–73.

86   discovery, joy, and delight: Todd Kashdan, *Curious? Discover the Missing Ingredient to a Fulfilling Life* (HarperCollins, 2009).

86   "I always wanted to know what was going to happen next": Rangan Chatterjee, "Auschwitz Survivor Dr. Edith Eger on How to Discover Your Inner Power," Dr. Chatterjee, January 1, 2021, https://drchatterjee.com/auschwitz-survivor-dr-edith-eger-on-how-to-discover-your-inner-power/.

86   curious people also have more satisfying relationships and marriages: Kashdan, *Curious?*

Week 22: Take a Silent Stroll

88   memory and learning: K. S Kraus. S. Mitra, et al., "Noise trauma impairs neurogenesis in the rat hippocampus," *Neuroscience* 167, no. 4 (June 2, 2010): 1216–26.

88   new neurons in their hippocampi: Imke Kirste, Zeina Nicola, et al., "Is silence golden? Effects of auditory stimuli and their absence on adult hippocampal neurogenesis," *Brain Structure & Function* 220, no. 2 (2015): 1221–28.

89   36 percent greater chance of getting Alzheimer's: Jennifer Weuve, Jennifer D'Souza, et al., "Long-term community noise exposure in relation to dementia, cognition, and cognitive decline in older adults." *Alzheimer's & Dementia* 17, no. 3 (March 2021): 525–33.

89   Even as we sleep: Harry Wallop, "How noise pollution affects your health—it takes years off your life," *The Sunday Times*, June 18, 2019, https://www.thetimes.co.uk/article/noise-pollution-isnt-just-annoying-it-affects-your-health-and-takes-years-off-your-life-q36rn2bvr.

89   dramatic effect on participants' stress markers: L. Bernardi, C. Porta, and P. Sleight, "Cardiovascular, cerebrovascular, and respiratory changes induced by different types of music in musicians and non-musicians: The importance of silence," *Heart* 92, no. 4 (April 2006): 445–52.

89   it *responds* to the silence: "Researchers find how brain hears the sound of silence," University of Oregon, February 10, 2010, https://uonews.uoregon.edu/archive/news-release/2010/2/researchers-find-how-brain-hears-sound-silence

90   between two strangers: Miao Cheng, Masaharu Kato, et al., "Paired walkers with better first impression synchronize better," *PLoS One*, February 21, 2020, DOI: doi.org/10.1371/journal.pone.0227880.

90   light was intensified by the lack of noise: Peter Matthiessen, *The Snow Leopard* (Vintage, 1998; originally published 1978).

Week 23: Walk at Altitude

93   than their sea-level peers: Majid Ezzati, Mara E. M. Horwitz, et al., "Altitude, life expectancy and mortality from ischaemic heart disease, stroke, COPD and cancers: national population-based analysis of US counties," *Journal of Epidemiology & Community Health* 66, no. 7 (2012): e17.

93   and exercise endurance improves: Rhea Maze, "A 17,000-foot view: CSU researcher finds surprising results in high-altitude study," Colorado State University

College News, July 27, 2018, https://cvmbs.source.colostate.edu/a-17000-foot-view-csu-researcher-finds-surprising-results-in-high-altitude-study/.

93–94   some conditions . . . less prevalent at higher altitude: Yanfei Guo, Zhenzhen Xing, et al., "Prevalence and risk factors for COPD at high altitude: A large cross-sectional survey of subjects living between 2,100–4,700 m above sea level," *Frontiers in Medicine* (Lausanne) 7 (2020): 581763.

94   repairing our cells and neurons in the process: Two of the many studies on this subject are: J. J. Larsen, J. M. Hansen, et al., "The effect of altitude hypoxia on glucose homeostasis in men," *Journal of Physiology* 504, no. 1 (1997): 241–49, and B. Kayser and S. Verges, "Hypoxia, energy balance and obesity: from pathophysiological mechanisms to new treatment strategies," *Obesity Reviews* 14, no. 7 (July 2013): 579–92.

94   avoiding the physiological stress of being at very high altitude: M. Burtscher, W. Nachbauer, et al., "Benefits of training at moderate altitude versus sea level training in amateur runners," *European Journal of Applied Physiology and Occupational Physiology* 74 (1996): 558–63.

Week 24: Walk with a Map

97   tarte Tatin in the evening: Sarah Hartley, *Mrs. P's Journey* (Simon & Schuster UK, 2001).

97   every London street: Eleanor A. Maguire, David G. Gadian, et al., "Navigation-related structural change in the hippocampi of taxi drivers," *Proceedings of the National Academy of Science of the USA* 97, no. 8 (April 11, 2000): 4398–403.

97   prone to Alzheimer's and dementia: Sarah Knapton, "Google Maps increases risk of developing Alzheimer's expert warns," *Telegraph*, May 29, 2019; https://www.telegraph.co.uk/science/2019/05/29/google-maps-increases-risk-developingalzheimers-expert-warns/.

98   navigate interpersonal relationships: Russell A. Epstein, Eva Zita Patel, et al., "The cognitive map in humans: Spatial navigation and beyond," *Nature Neuroscience* 20, no. 11 (October 26, 2017): 1504–13.

98   additional demands on the brain: Demands on the prefrontal cortex rather than the hippocampus. See Epstein et al., "The cognitive map in humans."

99   with staggering success: Brian Handwerk, "In Some Ways, Your Sense of Smell Is Actually Better Than a Dog's," *Smithsonian Magazine*, May 22, 2017, https://www.smithsonianmag.com/science-nature/you-actually-smell-better-dog-180963391/.

99   lichen can be used to orient ourselves: For instance, Tristan Gooley, *The Walker's Guide to Outdoor Clues and Signs* (Sceptre, 2014).

99   growing parental concerns with safety: Michael Bond, *Wayfinding: The Art and Science of How We Find and Lose Our Way* (Picador, 2020).

Week 25: Walk with Purpose

102 "walking for utilitarian purposes": Gilsu Pae and Gulsah Akar, "Effects of walking on self-assessed health status: Links between walking, trip purposes and health," *Journal of Transport & Health* 18 (September 2020): 100901.

103 much harder to procrastinate: Author interview, November 2020.

104 walk farther and for longer: David R. Bassett Jr. et al., "Step Counting: A Review of Measurement Considerations and Health-Related Applications," *Sports Medicine* 47, no. 7 (2017): 1303–15.

Week 26: Walk in Sunshine

105 "useful and important effect": Joseph S. Alpert, "The Jeremiah Metzger Lecture: Jeremiah Metzger and the Era of Heliotherapy," *Transactions of the American Clinical and Climatological Association* 126 (2015): 219–26.

106 "days of death and disease": *The Times*, quoted in Simon Carter, *Rise and Shine: Sunlight, Technology and Health* (Berg, 2007), 64.

106 five and thirty minutes of light: Lars Alfredsson, Bruce K. Armstrong, et al., "Insufficient sun exposure has become a real public health problem," *International Journal of Environmental Research and Public Health* 17, no. 14 (2020): 5014.

107 flu and common cold at bay: John Cannell et al., "On the epidemiology of influenza," *Virology Journal* 5, article no. 29 (2008). See also John Cannell et al., "Epidemic influenza and vitamin D," *Epidemiology and Infection* 134, no. 6 (2006): 1129–40.

107 numerous other studies: For example, Beata M. Gruber-Bzura, "Vitamin D and influenza—prevention or therapy?" *International Journal of Molecular Sciences* 19, no. 8 (2018): 2419.

107 dramatically higher rate of death among sun-avoiders: Marcia Frellick, "Avoiding sun as dangerous as smoking," Medscape, March 23, 2016, or P. G. Lindqvist, E. Epstein, et al., "Avoidance of sun exposure as a risk factor for major causes of death: A competing risk analysis of the melanoma in Southern Sweden cohort," *Journal of Internal Medicine* 280, no. 4 (2016): 375–87.

107 "effects of sun exposure": Jörg Reichrath, ed., *Sunlight, Vitamin D and Skin Cancer* (Springer, 2017), 120.

107 into our circulatory system: "Sunshine could benefit health and prolong life, study suggests," EurekAlert!, May 7, 2013, https://www.eurekalert.org/pub_releases/2013-05/uoe-scb050713.php.

107 "Sunlight directly activates key immune cells": Thieu X. Phan, Barbara Jaruga, et al., "Intrinsic photosensitivity enhances motility of T lymphocytes," *Nature Scientific Reports* 6, article no. 39479 (2016).

107 helping us to wake and sleep: H. J. van der Rhee, E. de Vries, and J. W. Coebergh, "Regular sun exposure benefits health," *Medical Hypotheses* 97 (2016): 34–37.

108 our microbiome: See, for instance, Dr. Tim Spector, "The sun goes down on vitamin D: Why I changed my mind about this celebrated supplement," The Conversation, January 6, 2016, https://theconversation.com/the-sun-goes-

down-on-vitamin-d-why-i-changed-my-mind-about-this-celebrated-supplement-52725.

108 "it intoxicates and poisons": Quoted in Elena Conis, "The Rise and Fall of Sunlight Therapy," *Los Angeles Times*, May 28, 2007.

108 risk of vitamin D deficiency: Farhad Hosseinpanah, Sima Hashemi pour, et al., "The effects of air pollution on vitamin D status in healthy women: A cross sectional study," *BMC Public Health* 10 (2010): 519.

109 a study in *The Lancet*: GW Lambert, PhD, et al., "Effect of Sunlight and Season on Serotonin Turnover in the Brain," *The Lancet* 360, no. 9348 (2002): 1840–42.

Week 27: Sing as You Stride

111 singing produces endorphins: Daisy Fancourt, Aaron Williamon, et al., "Singing modulates mood, stress, cortisol, cytokine and neuropeptide activity in cancer patients and carers," ecancer, April 5, 2016, https://ecancer.org/en/journal/article/631-singing-modulates-mood-stress-cortisol-cytokine-and-neuropeptide-activity-in-cancer-patients-and-carers/abstract.

112 choir and solo singing: T. Moritz Schladt, Gregory C. Nordmann, et al., "Choir versus solo singing: Effects on mood, and salivary oxytocin and cortisol concentrations," *Frontiers in Human Neuroscience* 11 (September 14, 2017): 430.

112 toward those we're singing with: "'Imperfect Harmony': How Singing with Others Changes Your Life," NPR, June 3, 2013, https://www.npr.org/2013/06/03/188355968/imperfect-harmony-how-chorale-singing-changes-lives.

112 dramatic results: Seung Yeol Lee, Hyun Seok, et al., "Immediate effects of mental singing while walking on gait disturbance in hemiplegic stroke patients: A feasibility study," *Annals of Rehabilitation Medicine* 42, no. 1 (2018): 1–7.

112 greater improvements than any other intervention: Elinor C. Harrison, Marie E. McNeely, and Gammon M. Earhart, "The feasibility of singing to improve gait in Parkinson disease," *Gait & Posture* 53 (2017): 224–29.

Week 28: Walk with a Picnic

114 "baskets of fresh fruit": Isabella Beeton, *Beeton's Book of Household Management* (1861).

115 concentric and eccentric contractions: N. Babault, M. Pousson, et al., "Activation of human quadriceps femoris during isometric, concentric, and eccentric contractions," *Journal of Applied Physiology* 91, no. 6 (2001): 2628–34.

116 "rocks, mountain heath and moss": Ellen Weeton, *Journal of a Governess, 1807–11* and *1811–25*.

116 sold at the local market: Gladys Mary Coles, *Mary Webb* (Seren Books, 1995).

116 weighed many pounds: Bill Laws, *Byways, Boots & Blisters: A History of Walkers & Walking* (The History Press, 2009).

117–18 if one arm only is used: Mike McRae, "Weight training in one arm has benefits for the other, even if it doesn't do a thing," Science Alert, October 25, 2020, https://www.sciencealert.com/weight-training-in-one-arm-has-benefits-for-the-other-one-even-if-it-doesn-t-lift-a-thing.

Week 29: Walk Barefoot

119 "evident to all who had seeing eyes": Society for Barefoot Living, https://www
.barefooters.org/the-barefoot-league/.

120 leaving us vulnerable to falls: Karen Weintraub, "Going Barefoot Is Good for the
Sole," *Scientific American*, June 26, 2019, https://www.scientificamerican.com
/article/going-barefoot-is-good-for-the-sole/.

120 healthier and better-formed feet: B. Zipfel, L. R. Berger, "Shod versus unshod: The
emergence of forefoot pathology in modern humans?" *The Foot* 17, no. 4 (2007)
205–13.

120 positively altered gait: Society for Barefoot Living, Medical Research, https://www
.barefooters.org/medical-research/.

120 "reduce the work that the foot muscles have to do": Freddy Sichting, Nicholas B.
Holowka, et al., "Effect of the upward curvature of toe springs on walking
biomechanics in humans," *Nature Scientific Reports* 10, article no. 14643 (2020).

121 strengthen the arches and muscles of our feet: Elizabeth E. Miller, Katherine
Whitcome, et al., "The effect of minimal shoes on arch structure and intrinsic foot
muscle strength," *Journal of Sport and Health Science* 3, no. 2 (2014): 74–85.

Week 30: Walk with Ions

122 "utterly Lord over us": All quotes from Samuel Taylor Coleridge and Robert
Macfarlane in this chapter from Macfarlane's *The Wild Places* (Granta, 2017),
207–10.

123 negative air ions: Negative air ions (NAIs) are sometimes called anions, and
positive air ions (PAIs) are sometimes called cations. NAIs carry an extra charge,
while PAIs lose one or more electrons.

123 *waterfall effect:* Shu-Ye Jiang, Ali Ma, and Srinivasan Ramachandran, "Negative air
ions and their effects on human health and air quality improvement," *International
Journal of Molecular Sciences* 19, no. 10 (2018): 2966.

123 up to 120 times higher than normal outdoor air: Predrag Kolarž, Martin Gaisberger,
et al., "Characterization of ions at Alpine waterfalls," *Atmospheric Chemistry and
Physics* 12, no. 8 (2012): 3687–97.

123 reduced their levels of inflammation: Martin Gaisberger, Renata Šanović, et al.,
"Effects of ionized waterfall aerosol on pediatric allergic asthma," *Journal of Asthma*
49, no. 8 (2012): 830–38.

124 waterfall group continued to show improved immunity: Carina Grafelstätter,
Martin Gaisberger, et al., "Does waterfall aerosol influence mucosal immunity and
chronic stress? A randomized controlled clinical trial," *Journal of Physiological
Anthropology* 36 (2017): 10.

125 negative air ions were capable of deactivating coronaviruses: Benjamin J. Scherlag,
Ronald A. Scherlag, and Sunny S. Po, "A potential non-invasive therapy to treat
COVID-19, as yet unrecognized in the medical literature," *International Archives
of Internal Medicine* 4, no. 2 (2020), https://clinmedjournals.org/articles/iaim
/international-archives-of-internal-medicine-iaim-4-027.pdf.

125 up to twenty minutes: Hui Wang, Bing Wang, et al., "Study on the change of negative air ion concentration and its influencing factors at different spatio-temporal scales," *Global Ecology and Conservation* 23 (2020): e01008.

125 NAIs linger in the air: Hui Wang, Bing Wang, et al., "Study on the change of negative air ion concentration and its influencing factors at different spatio-temporal scales."

126 Negative ions increase when rain falls: A. K. Kamra, A. S. Gautam, and Devendraa Siingh, "Charged nanoparticles produced by splashing of raindrops," *JGR: Atmospheres* 120, no. 13 (July 16, 2015): 6669–81.

126 maximize NAI exposure: Hui Wang, Bing Wang, et al., "Study on the change of negative air ion concentration."

Week 31: Walk Beside the Sea

128 "We are creatures of the ocean": Callum Roberts, *The Ocean of Life* (Penguin, 2013).

128 lowest-earning households: Joanne K. Garrett, Theodore J. Clitherow, et al., "Coastal proximity and mental health among urban adults in England: The moderating effect of household income," *Health & Place* 59 (September 2019): 102200.

128 experienced less depression: Seraphim Dempsey et al., "Coastal Blue Space and Depression in Older Adults," *Health & Place* 54 (2018): 110–117.

128 "natural restoration": Quoted in Wallace J. Nichols, *Blue Mind: How Water Makes You Happier, More Connected and Better at What You Do* (Abacus, 2014).

129 vortex of its own thoughts: Dr. Mathew White quoted in Elle Hunt, "Blue spaces: Why time spent near water is the secret of happiness," *The Guardian*, November 3, 2019, https://www.theguardian.com/lifeandstyle/2019/nov/03/blue-space-living-near-water-good-secret-of-happiness.

129 how often should we seek out the sea?: Anna Turns, "The Ocean Effect," *Coast*, January 2017, https://bluehealth2020.eu/wp/wp-content/uploads/2017/01/Coast_January-2017_BlueHealth.pdf.

Week 32: Walk in Water

130 attributed to lowered inflammation: Heather & Kandala Massey, et al., "Mood and Well-Being of Novice Open Water Swimmers and Controls During an Introductory Outdoor Swimming Programme: A Feasibility Study," *Journal of Lifestyle Medicine* 1 (2020).

132 recover their muscle and balance: Jae-Hyun Lee and Eunsook Sung, "The effects of aquatic walking and jogging program on physical function and fall efficacy in patients with degenerative lumbar spinal stenosis," *Journal of Exercise Rehabilitation* 11, no. 5 (2015): 272–75.

132 water walking raised the heart rate: A. Conti, C. Minganti, et al., "Cardiorespiratory of land and water walking on a non-motorized treadmill," *Journal of Sports Medicine and Physical Fitness* 55, no. 3 (2015): 179–84.

132 unfit women reduced their blood pressure: Daniel Rodriguez, Valter Silva, et al., "Hypotensive response after water-walking and land-walking exercise sessions in healthy trained and untrained women," *International Journal of General Medicine* 4 (2011): 549–54.

133 People with fibromyalgia who tried water walking: Hannah Denton and Kay Aranda, "The wellbeing benefits of sea swimming. Is it time to revisit the sea cure?" *Qualitative Research in Sport, Exercise and Health* 12, no. 5 (2020): 647–63.

133 submerged to the neck: Gravitational force is reduced by 30 percent at knee level, 50 percent at waist level, and 90 percent at neck level.

133 chest-deep water: Hyosok Lim, Daniel Azurdia, et al., "Influence of water depth on energy expenditure during aquatic walking in people post stroke," *Physiotherapy Research International* 23, no. 3 (2018): e1717.

Week 33: Sketch as You Walk

136 "less medication needed to induce sleep": Rosalia Lelchuk Staricoff, "Arts in health: The value of evaluation," *Journal of the Royal Society for the Promotion of Health* 126, no. 3 (2006): 116–20.

136 "visual art production has an impact": Anne Bolwerk, Jessica Mack-Andrick, et al., "How art changes your brain: Differential effects of visual art production and cognitive art evaluation on functional brain connectivity," *PLoS One* 9, no. 7 (2014): e101035.

136 creating art an excellent means of managing stress: Dafna Regev and Liat Cohen-Yatziv, "Effectiveness of art therapy with adult clients in 2018—what progress has been made?" *Frontiers in Psychology* 9 (2018): 1531.

137 those who started drawing and painting in midlife: Rosebud O. Roberts, Ruth H. Cha, et al., "Risk and protective factors for cognitive impairment in persons aged 85 years and older," *Neurology* 84, no. 18 (May 5, 2015): 1854–61.

Week 34: Walk Beneath a Full Moon

139 what my midwife had said: Ryotaro Wake, Takuya Misugi, et al., "The effect of the gravitation of the moon on frequency of births," *Environmental Health Insights* 4 (2010): 65–69.

140 "human sleep and evening melatonin levels": Christian Cajochen, Songül Altanay-Ekici, et al., "Evidence that the lunar cycle influences human sleep," *Current Biology* 23, no. 15 (2013): 1485–88.

140 at least three other reports: Ciro Della Monica, Giuseppe Atzori, and Derk-Jan Dijk, "Effects of lunar phase on sleep in men and women in Surrey," *Journal of Sleep Research* 24, no. 6 (2015): 687–94.

140 "association exists between moon phases and homicides": Simo Näyhä, "Lunar cycle in homicides: A population-based time series study in Finland," *BMJ Open* 9, no. 1 (2019): e022759.

140 "psychiatric emergencies decreased significantly": A. L. Lieber, "Human Aggression and the Lunar Synodic Cycle," National Criminal Justice Reference Service, 1978,

https://www.ojp.gov/ncjrs/virtual-library/abstracts/human-aggression-and-lunar-synodic-cycle.

141 higher numbers of female suicides: Victor Benno Meyer-Rochow, Tapani Hakko, et al., "Synodic lunar phases and suicide: Based on 2605 suicides over 23 years, a full moon peak is apparent in premenopausal women from northern Finland," *Molecular Psychiatry*, May 2020, DOI:10.1038/s41380-020-0768-7.

141 European badgers and domestic cattle: Florian Raible, Hiroki Takekata, and Kristin Tessmar-Raible, "An overview of monthly rhythms and clocks," *Frontiers in Neurology* 8 (2017): 189.

Week 35: Walk Like a Nomad

146 "quality of life, mood, and cognitive functioning": Kelsey T. Laird, Pattharee Paholpak, et al., "Mind-body therapies for late-life mental and cognitive health," *Current Psychiatry Reports* 20 (2018): article no. 2.

Week 36: Walk with a Pack

148 "To walk is truly to live": Alice Brown, *By Oak and Thorn: A Record of English Days* (1886).

149 more prone to heart disease and high blood pressure: "Human hearts evolved for endurance," *Science Daily*, September 16, 2019, https://www.sciencedaily.com/releases/2019/09/190916170120.htm.

149 something our bodies are uniquely suited to: Daniel Lieberman, *Exercised: The Science of Physical Activity, Rest and Health* (Penguin, 2020).

150 When we walk with weight on our back: Jim Pate, senior physiologist at the Center for Health & Human Performance, quoted in *Health* magazine, January 2020.

150 "effectively restored": Taylor J. Kelty, Todd R. Schachtman, et al., "Resistance-exercise training ameliorates LPS-induced cognitive impairment concurrent with molecular signaling changes in the rat dentate gyrus," *Journal of Applied Physiology* 127, no. 1 (2019): 254–63.

150 Stew Smith recommends: "Training for Ruck Marches," Stew Smith Fitness, http://www.stewsmith.com/linkpages/ruckmarches.htm.

150 "especially when sustained over time": Lisa Mosconi, *The XX Brain: The Groundbreaking Science Empowering Women to Prevent Dementia* (Allen & Unwin, 2020), 232.

151 90 percent of our muscles: Author interview with Martin Christie, March 2019.

152 vital when rucking: Author interview with Lieutenant Liam O'Kelly, December 20, 2020.

152 Take a friend: Simone Schnall, Kent D. Harber, et al., "Social support and the perception of geographical slant," *Journal of Experimental Social Psychology* 44, no. 5 (2008): 1246–55.

152 merely imagining a friend has the same effect: Schnall, Harber, et al., "Social support and the perception of geographical slant."

Week 37: Take a Foraging Walk

154 "weed lessons": Patience Gray, *Honey from a Weed* (Prospect Books, 2001).

154 hunter-gatherers in Tanzania: Alyssa N. Crittenden and David A. Zes, "Food sharing among Hadza hunter-gatherer children," *PLos One* 10, no. 7 (2015): e0131996.

154 top eleven superfoods: Anna Brooks, "15 Superfoods and the Scientific Reasons to Eat Them," Everyday Health, May 12, 2020, https://www.everydayhealth.com /photogallery/superfoods.aspx.

155 "greater short-term memory": Barbara Shukitt-Hale, Vivian Cheng, and James A. Joseph, "Effects of blackberries on motor and cognitive function in aged rats," *Nutritional Neuroscience* 12, no. 3 (2009): 135–40.

155 mycotherapy: Ivan V. Zmitrovich, Nina V. Belova, et al., "Cancer without pharmacological illusions and a niche for mycotherapy (review)," *International Journal of Medicinal Mushrooms* 21, no. 2 (2019): 105–19.

155 nettle tops: Mahmood Abedinzade, Mohammad Rostampour, et al., "Urtica Dioica and Lamium Album decrease glycogen synthase kinase-3 beta and increase K-Ras in diabetic rats," *Journal of Pharmacopuncture* 22, no. 4 (2019): 248–52.

155 wild garlic: Roman Leontiev, Nils Hohaus, et al., "A comparison of the antibacterial and antifungal activities of thiosulfinate analogues of allicin," *Nature Scientific Reports* 8, article no. 6763 (2018). https://www.nature.com/articles/s41598-018-25154-9.

155 a daily handful of nuts: "Eating nuts can lower cholesterol, say experts," BBC News, May 10, 2010, http://news.bbc.co.uk/1/hi/health/8673208.stm.

156 curbed our cravings: "Short walk cuts chocolate consumption in half," Research News, University of Exeter, December 7, 2011.

Week 38: Climb Hills

157 "the exertion of the ascent": Quoted in Duncan Minshull, ed., *The Vintage Book of Walking* (Vintage, 2000).

158 movement in a long climb: Nan Shepherd, *The Living Mountain* (Canongate, 2011; first published 1977).

158 when we walk uphill: J. R. Franz, R. Kram, "The Effects of Grade and Speed on Leg Muscle Activations During Walking," *Gait Posture* 35, no. 1 (2012):143–47.

159 downhill walking might be an excellent option: Marc Phillippe, Hannes Gatterer, et al., "The effects of 3 weeks of uphill and downhill walking on blood lipids and glucose metabolism in pre-diabetic men: A pilot study," *Journal of Sports Science & Medicine* 16, no. 1 (2017): 35–43.

160 "these minor evils": Clare Roche, "Women climbers 1850–1900: A challenge to male hegemony?" *Sport in History* 33, no. 3 (2013): 236–59.

160 tiredness on long ascents: Nicola Giovanelli, Michele Sulli, et al., "Do poles save energy during steep uphill walking?" *European Journal of Applied Physiology* 119, no. 7 (2019): 1557–63.

160 include uphill walking: Clarissa S. Whiting, Stephen P. Allen, et al., "Steep (30°) uphill walking vs. running: COM movements, stride kinematics, and leg muscle excitations," *European Journal of Applied Physiology* 120, no. 10 (2020): 2147–57.

160 Take a friend: Simone Schnall, Kent D. Harber, et al., "Social support and the perception of geographical slant," *Journal of Experimental Social Psychology* 44, no. 5 (2008): 1246–55.

Week 39: Walk with Your Nose

161 "the hours of a July day": Rachel Carson, "An Island I Remember," *Lost Woods: The Discovered Writing of Rachel Carson* (Beacon Press, 1999).

162 antiseptic, anticarcinogenic, and antifungal: Hazem S. Elshafie and Ippolito Camele, "An overview of the biological effects of some Mediterranean essential oils on human health," Bioactive Natural Products 2017, https://www.hindawi.com/journals/bmri/2017/9268468/.

162 arrest the proliferation of cancer cells: Bing Qui, Wei Jiang, et al., "Pine needle oil induces G2/M arrest of HepG2 cells by activating the ATM pathway," *Experimental and Therapeutic Medicine* 15, no. 2 (2018): 1975–81.

162 could help suppress tumors: Nguyen Thi Hoai, Ho Viet Duc, et al. "Selectivity of *Pinus sylvestris* extract and essential oil to estrogen-insensitive breast cancer cells *Pinus sylvestris* against cancer cells," *Pharmacognosy Magazine* 11, suppl. 2 (2015): S290–S295.

163 inhaling rosemary oil: See, for instance, Mahboobeh Ghasemzadeh Rahbardar, Bahareh Amin, et al., "Anti-inflammatory effects of ethanolic extract of Rosmarinus officinalis L. and rosmarinic acid in a rat model of neuropathic pain," *Biomedicine & Pharmacotherapy* 86 (2017): 441–49. A 2019 study claimed that rosemary's phenolic compounds "had a profound effect on inflammation and inflammatory mediators." Mahboobeh Ghasemzadeh Rahbardar, Bahareh Amin, et al., "Rosmarinic acid attenuates development and existing pain in a rat model of neuropathic pain: An evidence of anti-oxidative and anti-inflammatory effects," *Phytomedicine* 40 (2018): 59–67.

163 "lavender inhalation can significantly reduce anxiety levels": Davide Donelli, Michele Antonelli, et al., "Effects of lavender on anxiety: A systematic review and meta-analysis," *Phytomedicine* 65 (2019): 153099.

163 improve feelings of relaxation: Kathryn Shady, Julie M. Nair, and Courtney Crannell, "Lavender aromatherapy: Examining the effects of lavender oil patches on patients in the hematology-oncology setting," *Clinical Journal of Oncology Nursing* 23, no. 5 (2019): 502–508.

163 deeper sleep and improved concentration: Kandhasamy Sowndhararajan and Songmun Kim, "Influence of fragrances on human psychophysiological activity: With special reference to human electroencephalographic response," *Scientia Pharmaceutica* 84, no. 4 (2016): 724–52.

163 peppermint oil has successfully curbed nausea and vomiting: Carla Mohr, Cassandra Jensen, et al., "Peppermint essential oil for nausea and vomiting in

hospitalized patients: Incorporating holistic patient decision making into the research design," *Journal of Holistic Nursing*, September 27, 2020, DOI: 10.1177 /0898010120961579.

163 sage oil dramatically slows the pulse rates: Milena Mitic, Adrijana Zrnič, et al., "Clary sage essential oil and its effect on human mood and pulse rate: An in vivo pilot study," *Planta Medica* 86, no. 15 (2020): 1125–32.

Week 40: Walk Like a Pilgrim

165 her deep spirituality: Rebecca Solnit, *Wanderlust: A History of Walking* (Granta, 2014).

166 Three hundred and thirty million people: Clare Gogerty, *Beyond the Footpath: Mindful Adventures for Modern Pilgrims* (Piatkus, 2019).

167 "a new awareness": Nancy Louise Frey, *Pilgrim Stories: On and Off the Road to Santiago* (University of California Press, 1998).

167 "the here and now": Frey, *Pilgrim Stories.*

167 "pronounced shifts in perception": Bill Hathaway, "Where the brain processes spiritual experiences," Yale News, May 29, 2018, https://news.yale.edu/2018/05 /29/where-brain-processes-spiritual-experiences.

167 a sense of the spiritual promoted higher levels of life satisfaction: Irini Gergianaki, Maria Kampouraki, et al., "Assessing spirituality: Is there a beneficial role in the management of COPD?" *npj Primary Care Respiratory Medicine* 29, article no. 23 (2019).

167 "things that can increase mortality": Marino A. Bruce, David Martins, et al., "Church attendance, allostatic load and mortality in middle aged adults," *PLoS One* 12, no. 5 (2017): e0177618.

167 spiritual experience linked to raised levels of multiple neurochemicals: E. Mohandas, "Neurobiology of Spirituality," *Mens Sana Monographs* 6, no. 1 (2008): 63–80.

168 "most women need to exercise for longer periods at lower intensity": Lisa Mosconi, *The XX Brain: The Groundbreaking Science Empowering Women to Prevent Dementia* (Allen & Unwin, 2020).

169 in the footsteps of Harriet Tubman: Kate Torgovnick May, "What we learned from walking in the footsteps of Harriet Tubman," Ideas.TED.com, January 17, 2019, https://ideas.ted.com/what-we-learned-from-walking-in-the-footsteps-of-harriet-tubman/.

Week 41: Walk to Get Lost

170 psychological response to the landscape: Guy Debord, "Theory of the Dérive," *Les Lèvres Nues,* no. 9, November 1956, https://www.cddc.vt.edu/sionline/si/theory .html.

171 place and grid cells atrophied: Kyle T. Gagnon, Elizabeth A. Cashdan, et al., "Sex differences in exploration behavior and the relationship to harm avoidance," *Human Nature* 27 (2016): 82–97.

172 as little as fifteen hours: More information on Sorby and the training course she developed can be found here: "Spatial skills are building blocks to STEM success," Ohio State University College of Engineering, February 29, 2016, https://engineering.osu.edu/news/2016/02/spatial-skills-are-building-blocks-stem-success.

172 Debord's *Theory of the Dérive*: https://www.cddc.vt.edu/sionline/si/theory.html.

Week 42: Walk After Eating

174 "transit time was dramatically accelerated": G. J. Oettlé, "Effect of moderate exercise on bowel habit," *Gut* 32, no. 8 (1991): 941–44.

174 "total colonic transit time": Anneke M. De Schryver, Yolande C. Keulemans, et al., "Effects of regular physical activity on defecation pattern in middle-aged patients complaining of chronic constipation," *Scandinavian Journal of Gastroenterology* 40, no. 4 (2005): 422–29.

174 reduce the need for insulin injections: Andrew N. Reynolds, Jim I. Mann, et al., "Advice to walk after meals is more effective for lowering postprandial glycaemia in type 2 diabetes mellitus than advice that does not specify timing: A randomised crossover study," *Diabetologia* 59, no. 12 (2016): 2572–78.

174 "beneficial impact on postprandial glycemia": Marah Aqeel, Anna Forster, et al., "The effect of timing of exercise and eating on postprandial response in adults: A systematic review," *Nutrients* 12, no. 1 (2020): 221.

175 three ten-minute walks may be more effective: S. Park, L. D. Rink, and J. P Wallace, "Accumulation of physical activity: Blood pressure reduction between 10-min walking sessions," *Journal of Human Hypertension* 22, no. 7 (2008): 475–82.

Week 43: Walk with Others

177 "a profoundly social activity": Tim Ingold and Jo Lee Vergunst, eds., *Ways of Walking: Ethnography and Practice on Foot,* Anthropological Studies of Creativity and Perception series (Ashgate, 2008).

178 Merely shaking hands: Maria Cohut, "What are the health benefits of being social?" *Medical News Today*, February 23, 2018, https://www.medicalnewstoday.com/articles/321019#Why-are-we-a-social-species?

178 good social ties: Annabel Streets and Susan Saunders, *The Age-Well Project: Easy Ways to a Longer, Healthier, Happier Life*, London (Piatkus, 2019).

178 three times more likely to develop depression: Maria Elizabeth Loades, Eleanor Chatburn, et al., "Rapid systematic review: The impact of social isolation and loneliness on the mental health of children and adolescents in the context of COVID-19," *Journal of the American Academy of Child & Adolescent Psychiatry* 59, no. 11 (2020): P1218–1239.e3.

178 loneliness is as damaging as smoking: Streets and Saunders, *The Age-Well Project*, 207.

178 low dropout rates: Catherine Meads and Josephine Exley, "A systematic review of group walking in physically healthy people to promote physical activity," *International Journal of Technology Assessment in Health Care* 34, no. 1 (January 17, 2018): 27–37.

179 drop in feelings of stress and depression: Tessa M. Pollard, Cornelia Guell, and Stephanie Morris, "Communal therapeutic mobility in group walking: A meta-ethnography," *Social Science and Medicine* 262 (October 2020): 113241.

179 acceptance, belonging and safety: Interview with the author, November 2020.

180 regular walks often became lifelines: Stephanie Morris, Cornelia Guell, and Tessa M. Pollard, "Group walking as a 'lifeline': Understanding the place of outdoor walking groups in women's lives," *Social Science & Medicine* 238 (October 2019): 112489.

180 hunted in pairs: Daniel Lieberman, *Exercised: The Science of Physical Activity, Rest and Health* (Penguin, 2020).

180 "but a stepping stone to recovery": Melissa R. Marselle, Sara L. Warber, and Katherine N. Irvine, "Growing resilience through interaction with nature: Can group walks in nature buffer the effects of stressful life events on mental health?" *International Journal of Environmental Research and Public Health* 16, no. 6 (2019): 986.

180 "emotional rescue": Ralf Buckley and Diane Westaway, "Mental health rescue effects of women's outdoor tourism: A role in COVID-19 recovery," *Annals of Tourism Research* 85 (November 2020): 103041.

181 "it's better to go alone": Florence Williams, *The Nature Fix: Why Nature Makes Us Happier, Healthier, and More Creative* (W. W. Norton, 2017), 167.

Week 44: Seek Out the Sublime

183 dropped jaws: Michelle N. Shiota, Belinda Campos, and Dacher Keltner, "The faces of positive emotion: Prototype displays of awe, amusement, and pride," *Annals of the New York Academy of Sciences* 1000 (2003): 296–99.

183 When she exposed individuals to awe: Melanie Rudd, Kathleen Vohs, and Jennifer Aaker, "Awe expands people's perception of time, alters decision making, and enhances well-being," *Psychological Science* 23, no. 10 (2012): 1130–36.

184 better able to deal with uncertainty: Paul K. Piff et al., "Awe, the small self, and prosocial behavior," *Journal of Personality and Social Psychology* 108, no. 6 (2015): 883–99.

184 and with depression: Raised levels of IL-6 are so prevalent in the blood of the severely depressed, they've become known as a biological suicide marker. See V. A. L. Miná, S. F. Lacerda-Pinheiro, et al., "The influence of inflammatory cytokines in physiopathology of suicidal behavior," *Journal of Affective Disorders* 172 (2015): 219–30.

184 the lowest levels of IL-6: Jennifer E. Stellar, Neha John-Henderson, et al., "Positive affect and markers of inflammation: Discrete positive emotions predict lower levels of inflammatory cytokines," *Emotion* 15, no. 2 (2015): 129–33.

184 the greater our potential well-being: Nicholas Weiler, "'Awe Walks' Boost Emotional Well-Being," University of California San Francisco, September 21, 2020, https://www.ucsf.edu/news/2020/09/418551/awe-walks-boost-emotional-well-being.

185 more likely to experience the sublime: Craig L. Anderson, Dante D. Dixson, et al., "Are awe-prone people more curious? The relationship between dispositional awe, curiosity, and academic outcomes," *Journal of Personality* 88, no. 4 (2020): 762–79.

Week 45: Work as You Walk

187 deskercisers: Kayla M. Frodsham, Nicholas R. Randall, et al., "Does type of active workstation matter? A randomized comparison of cognitive and typing performance between rest, cycling, and treadmill active workstations," *PLoS One* 15, no. 8 (2020): e0237348.

187 brain parts associated with memory and attention: Élise Labonté-LeMoyne, Radhika Santhanam, et al., "The delayed effect of treadmill desk usage on recall and attention," *Computers in Human Behavior* 46 (May 2015): 1–5.

188 reducing the number of errors: Gordon Dodwell, Hermann J. Müller, and Thomas Töllner, "Electroencephalographic evidence for improved visual working memory performance during standing and exercise," *British Journal of Psychology* 110, no. 2 (May 2019): 400–27.

188 more ideas while walking: M. Oppezzo and D. L. Schwartz, "Give your ideas some legs: The positive effect of walking on creative thinking," *Journal of Experimental Psychology: Learning, Memory, and Cognition* 40, no. 4 (2014): 1142–52.

188 new ideas in greater quantity: Christian Rominger, Andreas Fink, et al., "Everyday bodily movement is associated with creativity independently from active positive affect: A Bayesian mediation analysis approach," *Nature Scientific Reports* 10, article no. 11985 (2020).

188 facilitate lateral thought: Shane O'Mara, *In Praise of Walking: The New Science of How We Walk and Why It's Good for Us* (Penguin, 2019).

188 "enhances creative fluency": Shu Imaizumi, Ubuka Tagami, and Yi Yang, "Fluid movements enhance creative fluency: A replication of Slepian and Ambady (2012)," *PloS One* 15, no. 7 (July 30, 2020): e0236825. https://pubmed.ncbi.nlm.nih.gov/32730311/.

189 a walk should be taken outside: Oppezzo and Schwartz, "Give your ideas some legs."

Week 46: Take a Night Walk

191 equally important: Interview with the author, November 2020.

191 higher risk of developing breast cancer: Ron Chepesiuk, "Missing the dark: Health effects of light pollution," *Environmental Health Perspectives* 117, no. 1 (2009): A20–A27.

191 "interfere with normal brain cell structures": Eva M. Selhub and Alan C. Logan, *Your Brain on Nature: The Science of Nature's Influence on Your Health, Happiness, and Vitality* (Collins, 2014).

191 "to survive and thrive": Rachael Davies, "Why 'star walking' is the outdoor activity we need right now," *National Geographic*, March 10, 2021; American Medical Association Council on Science and Public Health (2012).

192 Take a UV flashlight: Heather Buttivant, *Rock Pool: Extraordinary Encounters Between the Tides* (September Publishing, 2019).

193 Dark Sky–accredited site: You can find them here: https://darksky.net.

Week 47: Jump-Start Your Walk for Super-Strong Bones

196 55 percent of Americans: International Osteoporosis Foundation, Facts and Statistics, https://www.osteoporosis.foundation/facts-statistics.

196 or more slowly: Diane Feskanich, Walter Willett, and Graham Colditz, "Walking and leisure-time activity and risk of hip fracture in postmenopausal women," *JAMA* 288, no. 18 (2002): 2300–306.

196 after a mere two months: J. Eric Strong, "Effects of Different Jumping Programs on Hip and Spine Bone Mineral Density in Pre-Menopausal Women," Brigham Young University Theses and Dissertations, February 2, 2004, https://scholarsarchive.byu.edu/cgi/viewcontent.cgi?article=1666&context=etd.

197 just about everyone: See for instance Dimitris Vlachopoulos, Alan R. Barker, et al., "The effect of a high-impact jumping intervention on bone mass, bone stiffness and fitness parameters in adolescent athletes," *Archives of Osteoporosis* 13, no. 1 (2018): 128, and Pamela S. Hinton, Peggy Nigh, and John Thyfault, "Effectiveness of resistance training or jumping-exercise to increase bone mineral density in men with low bone mass: A 12-month randomized, clinical trial," *Bone* 79 (2015): 203–12.

197 on a par with high jumpers: R. Nikander, P. Kannus, et al., "Targeted exercises against hip fragility," *Osteoporosis International* 20, no. 8 (2009): 1321–28.

197 bone density in the elderly: Pim Pellikaan, Georgios Giarmatzis, et al., "Ranking of osteogenic potential of physical exercises in postmenopausal women based on femoral neck strains," *PLoS One* 13, no. 4 (2018): e0195463.

198 incidence of hip fractures: Claire Chevalier, Silas Kieser, et al., "Warmth prevents bone loss through the gut microbiota," *Cell Metabolism* 32, no. 4 (2020): 575–590.e7.

198 caffeine aided and enhanced jumping: Nanci S. Guest, Trisha A. VanDusseldorp, et al., "International society of sports nutrition position stand: Caffeine and exercise performance," *Journal of the International Society of Sports Nutrition* 18, no. 1 (2021): 1.

198 prevent bone loss in their old age: A. Andreoli, M. Celi, et al., "Long-term effect of exercise on bone mineral density and body composition in post-menopausal ex-elite athletes: A retrospective study," *European Journal of Clinical Nutrition* 66, no. 1 (2012): 69–74.

Week 48: Walk Hungry

199 healthy young men who exercised before breakfast consumed less food: Robert M. Edinburgh, Aaron Hengist, et al., "Skipping breakfast before exercise creates a more negative 24-hour energy balance: A randomized controlled trial in healthy physically active young men," *Journal of Nutrition* 149, no. 8 (2019): 1326–34.

200 "positive and profound": Robert M. Edinburgh et al., "Lipid Metabolism Links Nutrient-Exercise Timing to Insulin Sensitivity in Men Classified as Overweight or Obese," *The Journal of Clinical Endocrinology & Metabolism* 105, no. 3 (2020): 660–76.

200 movement before breakfast may help curb inflammation: Edgars Liepinsh, Elina Makarova, et al., "Low-intensity exercise stimulates bioenergetics and increases fat oxidation in mitochondria of blood mononuclear cells from sedentary adults," *Physiological Reports* 8, no. 12 (June 2020): e14489.

201 fasted walking is particularly effective for reducing obesity: Pamela M. Peeke, Frank L. Greenway, et al., "Effect of time restricted eating on body weight and fasting glucose in participants with obesity: Results of a randomized, controlled, virtual clinical trial," *Nutrition & Diabetes* 11, no. 1 (2021): 6.

Week 49: Walk Backward

203 "good for health": Ben Montgomery, *The Man Who Walked Backward: An American Dreamer's Search for Meaning in the Great Depression* (Little, Brown, 2018).

203 different team of core and lower body muscles: Oluwole O. Awosika, Saira Matthews, et al., "Backward locomotor treadmill training combined with transcutaneous spinal direct current stimulation in stroke: A randomized pilot feasibility and safety study," *Brain Communications* 2, no. 1 (2020): fcaa045.

204 benefits our posture: Chet R. Whitley and Janet S. Dufek, "Effects of backward walking on hamstring flexibility and low back range of motion," *International Journal of Exercise Science* 4, no. 3 (2011).

204 reduced lower back pain: Janet Dufek, Anthony House, et al., "Backward walking: A possible active exercise for low back pain reduction and enhanced function in athletes," *Journal of Exercise Physiology Online* 14, no. 2 (2011): 17–26.

204 improved speed, stride, and gait: Hyun-Gyu Cha, Tae-Hoon Kim, and Myoung-Kwon Kim, "Therapeutic efficacy of walking backward and forward on a slope in normal adults," *Journal of Physical Therapy Science* 28, no. 6 (2016): 1901–3.

204 fewer mistakes in their subsequent work: Davide Viggiano, Michele Travaglio, et al., "Effect of backward walking on attention: Possible application on ADHD," *Translational Medicine @UniSa* 11 (December 19, 2014): 48–54.

206 easier to learn and remember: "Using Failures, Movement & Balance to Learn Faster," Huberman Lab Podcast #7, https://www.youtube.com/watch?v=hx3U64IXFOY.

Week 50: Walk in an Evergreen Forest (for a Good Night's Sleep)

207 "history of my own heart": Mary Wollstonecraft, *Letters Written During a Short Residence in Sweden, Norway, and Denmark* (1796).

208 the cleanest air we will ever breathe: Peter Wohlleben, *The Hidden Life of Trees* (William Collins, 2016).

208 rats to sleep for longer: Sadao Yamaoka, Teruyo Tomita, et al., "Effects of plant-derived odors on sleep–wakefulness and circadian rhythmicity in rats," *Chemical Senses* 30, suppl. 1(2005): i264—i265.

209 sleeping for longer: Hyeyun Kim, Yong Won Lee, et al., "An exploratory study on the effects of forest therapy on sleep quality in patients with gastrointestinal tract cancers," *International Journal of Environmental Research and Public Health* 16, no. 14 (2019): 2449.

209 the afternoon walkers: Emi Morita, Makato Imai, et al., "A before and after comparison of the effects of forest walking on the sleep of a community-based sample of people with sleep complaints," *BioPsychoSocial Medicine* 5, no. 1 (2011): 13.

209 the concentration of phytoncides will be at its highest: Qing Li, *Shinrin-Yoku: The Art and Science of Forest Bathing* (Penguin, 2018).

210 wind always disperses terpenes: Jaeseok Lee, Kyoung Sang Cho, et al., "Characteristics and distribution of terpenes in South Korean forests," *Journal of Ecology and Environment* 41, article no. 19 (2017).

210 peaked at four hours: Liisa Anderse, Sus Sola Corazon, and Ulrika Karlsson Stigsdotter, "Nature exposure and its effects on immune system functioning: A systematic review," *International Journal of Environmental Research and Public Health* 18, no. 4 (2021): 1416.

Week 51: Walking as Meditation

210 nightly sleep by forty-five minutes: K. G. Baron et al., "Exercise to Improve Sleep in Insomnia: Exploration of the Bidirectional Effects," *Journal of Clinical Sleep Medicine* 9, no. 8 (2013): 819–24.

212 "plagued by stress and burnout": Pamela van der Riet, Tracy Levett-Jones, and Catherine Aquino-Russell, "The effectiveness of mindfulness meditation for nurses and nursing students: An integrated literature review," *Nurse Education Today* 65 (2018): 201–11.

212 "improving [our] immune system, metabolism, and stress-response pathways": Sabrina Venditti, Loredana Verdone, et al., "Molecules of silence: Effects of meditation on gene expression and epigenetics," *Frontiers in Psychology* 11 (2020): 1767.

212 denser gray matter: Britta K. Hölzel, James Carmody, et al., "Mindfulness practice leads to increases in regional brain gray matter density," *Psychiatry Research: Neuroimaging* 191, no. 1 (January 30, 2011): 36–43.

213 as people half their age: "Welcome to the Lazar Lab," https://scholar.harvard.edu/sara_lazar/home, and Sue McGreevey, "Eight weeks to a better brain," *Harvard Gazette,* January 21, 2011, https://news.harvard.edu/gazette/story/2011/01/eight-weeks-to-a-better-brain/.

213 walking meditation reduced depression: Susaree Prakhinkit, Siriluck Suppapitiporn, et al., "Effects of Buddhism walking meditation on depression, functional fitness, and endothelium-dependent vasodilation in depressed elderly," *Journal of Alternative and Complementary Medicine* 20, no. 5 (2014): 411–16.

213 better balance and coordination: Apsornsawan Chatutain, Jindarut Pattana, et al., "Walking meditation promotes ankle proprioception and balance performance among elderly women," *Journal of Bodywork and Movement Therapies* 23, no. 3 (2019): 652–57.

213 rhythm of our steps: Sylvia Boorstein, *Don't Just Do Something, Sit There* (HarperCollins, 1996), p. 65.

214 improving our respiration and our circulation: Thich Nhat Hanh, "Walk Like a Buddha," *Tricycle*, summer 2011, https://tricycle.org/magazine/walk-buddha/.

215 lower back pain or anxiety: Meghan K. Edwards, Simon Rosenbaum, and Paul D. Loprinzi, "Differential experimental effects of a short bout of walking, meditation, or combination of walking and meditation on state anxiety among young adults," *American Journal of Health Promotion* 32, no. 4 (2018): 949–58; Anna M. Polaski, Amy L. Phelps, et al., "Integrated meditation and exercise therapy: A randomized controlled pilot of a combined nonpharmacological intervention focused on reducing disability and pain in patients with chronic low back pain," *Pain Medicine* 22, no. 2 (2021): 444–58.

Week 52: Walk Deep and Seek Fractals

216 "enriched and refreshed": Tony Hiss, *In Motion: The Experience of Travel* (Knopf, 2010).

217 our ability to focus: Julian Smith, Conor Rowland, et al., "Relaxing floors: Fractal fluency in the built environment," *Nonlinear Dynamics, Psychology and Life Sciences* 24, no. 1 (2020): 127–41.

217 reduce our stress levels by 60 percent: R. P. Taylor, "Reduction of physiological stress using fractal art and architecture," *Leonardo* 39, no. 3 (2006): 245–51.

218 deeply relaxing: Kelly E. Robles, Nicole A. Liaw, et al., "A shared fractal aesthetic across development," *Humanities and Social Sciences Communications* 7, article no. 158 (2020).

218 we can benefit merely from having fractals around us: For more on fractals, see Florence Williams, *The Nature Fix: Why Nature Makes Us Happier, Healthier, and More Creative* (W. W. Norton, 2017).

219 "shallow investigations": "Brain Mechanism of Curiosity Unraveled," *Neuroscience News*, May 13, 2021.

219 "full of possibility": Hiss, *In Motion*.

recommended reading

Abbs, Annabel. *Windswept: Walking the Paths of Trailblazing Women.* Portland: Tin House, 2021.

Andrews, Kerri. *Wanderers: A History of Women Walking.* London: Reaktion, 2020.

Elkin, Lauren. *Flâneuse: Women Walk the City in Paris, New York, Tokyo, Venice and London.* London: Chatto & Windus, 2016.

Geddes, Linda. *Chasing the Sun: The New Science of Sunlight and How It Shapes Our Bodies and Minds.* London: Wellcome Collection, 2019.

Godwin, Fay, and Shirley Toulson. *The Drovers' Roads of Wales.* London: Wildwood House, 1977.

Gogerty, Clare. *Beyond the Footpath: Mindful Adventures for Modern Pilgrims.* London: Piatkus, 2019.

Humble, Kate. *Thinking on My Feet: The Small Joy of Putting One Foot in Front of Another.* London: Aster, 2018.

Jebb, Miles. *Walkers.* London: Constable, 1985.

Kagge, Erling. *Walking: One Step at a Time*, trans. Becky L. Crook. London: Viking Press, 2019.

Laws, Bill. *Byways, Boots & Blisters: A History of Walkers & Walking.* Stroud, UK: The History Press, 2009.

Li, Qing. *Shinrin-Yoku: The Art and Science of Forest Bathing.* London: Penguin, 2018.

Lieberman, Daniel. *Exercised: The Science of Physical Activity, Rest and Health.* London: Penguin, 2021.

Nestor, James. *Breath: The New Science of a Lost Art.* London: Penguin Life, 2020.

Nicholson, Geoff. *The Lost Art of Walking: The History, Science, Philosophy, Literature, Theory and Practice of Pedestrianism.* Newmarket: Harbour Books, 2010.

Malchik, Antonia. *A Walking Life: Reclaiming Our Health and Our Freedom One Step at a Time.* New York: Da Capo, 2019.

Minshull, Duncan, ed. *While Wandering: A Walking Companion.* London: Vintage, 2014.

———, ed. *Beneath My Feet: Writers on Walking*, London: Notting Hill Editions, 2018.

————, ed. *Sauntering: Writers Walk Europe*. London: Notting Hill Editions, 2021.

Montgomery, Ben. *Grandma Gatewood's Walk: The Inspiring Story of the Woman Who Saved the Appalachian Trail*. Chicago: Chicago Review Press, 2016.

————. *The Man Who Walked Backward: An American Dreamer's Search for Meaning in the Great Depression*. New York: Little, Brown Spark, 2018.

Nichols, Wallace J. *Blue Mind: How Water Makes You Happier, More Connected and Better at What You Do*. London: Abacus, 2018.

O'Mara, Shane. *In Praise of Walking: The New Science of How We Walk and Why It's Good for Us*. London: Bodley Head, 2019.

Selhub, Eva M., and Alan C. Logan. *Your Brain on Nature: The Science of Nature's Influence on Your Health, Happiness, and Vitality*. London: Collins, 2014.

Shepherd, Nan. *The Living Mountain*. Edinburgh: Canongate, 2011.

Solnit, Rebecca. *Wanderlust: A History of Walking*. London: Granta, 2014.

Strayed, Cheryl. *Wild: A Journey from Lost to Found*. London: Atlantic, 2012.

Streets, Annabel, and Susan Saunders. *The Age-Well Project: Easy Ways to a Longer, Healthier, Happier Life*. London: Piatkus, 2019.

Sullivan, Danny. *Ley Lines: The Greatest Landscape Mystery*. Langport UK: Green Magic, 2004.

Walker, Peter. *The Miracle Pill: Why a Sedentary World Is Getting It All Wrong*. London: Simon & Schuster UK, 2021.

Williams, Florence. *The Nature Fix: Why Nature Makes Us Happier, Healthier, and More Creative*. New York: W. W. Norton, 2017.

————. *The 3-Day Effect*. Read by the author, Audible Original, 2019.

Wohlleben, Peter. *The Hidden Life of Trees: What They Feel, How They Communicate—Discoveries from a Secret World*. trans. Jane Billinghurst. London: William Collins, 2017.

————. *Walks in the Wild: A Guide Through the Forest*, trans. Ruth Ahmedzai Kemp. London: Rider, 2019.

index

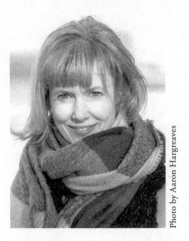

Photo by Aaron Hargreaves

ANNABEL STREETS is a writer of highly researched, award-winning fiction as well as both narrative and practical nonfiction. She is author, writing as Annabel Abbs, of the nonfiction book *Windswept: Walking the Paths of Trailblazing Women* (Tin House, 2021), a feminist meditation on the power of walking in the lives of several extraordinary women, including Georgia O'Keeffe, Simone de Beauvoir, and Frieda Lawrence. Under the name Annabel Streets, which she uses for her practical nonfiction, she is a coauthor of *The Age-Well Project* (Piatkus, 2019). She is the author of the novels *The Joyce Girl* (William Morrow, 2020), the story of James Joyce's daughter Lucia; *Frieda: The Original Lady Chatterley* (John Murray, 2018); and *Miss Eliza's English Kitchen* (William Morrow, 2021), which has been described as a *Julie & Julia* set in Victorian England. Her work has been translated into more than twenty languages.

CONNECT ONLINE

AnnabelAbbs.com

AgeWellProject.com

AbbsAnnabel

AnnabelAbbs